COVID19 AND THE CITY

THE COVID19 PANDEMIC AND THE TRANSFORMATION OF THE CITY

MARK J NIEUWENHUIJSEN, ISGLOBAL, BARCELONA, SPAIN

ISBN: 9798553841249

MJN Publishers, Barcelona, Spain

ABOUT THE AUTHOR

Mark J Nieuwenhuijsen PhD is a Research Professor and a director of Urban Planning, Environment and Health at the Institute for Global Health (ISGlobal), Barcelona, Spain and is a world leading expert in environmental exposure assessment, epidemiology, and health impact assessment with a strong focus and interest on healthy urban living.

He has edited 3 books on Exposure Assessment and on Environmental Epidemiology, and 1 on Integrating human health into Urban and Transport planning, 1 on Transportation and Health, 1 on Traffic Related Air Pollution and has co-authored more than 450 papers published in peer reviewed journals and 35 book chapters. In 2018, he was awarded the ISEE John Goldsmith Award for Outstanding Contributions to Environmental Epidemiology. In both 2018 and 2019 he was among the 1% most cited scientists in the world.

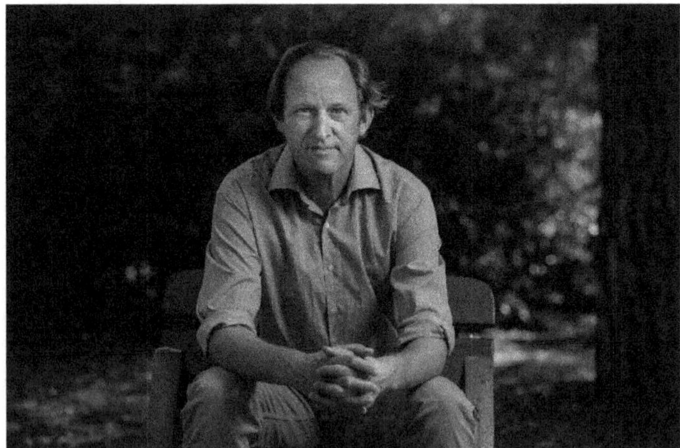

©Jordi Play

Address correspondence to

Mark J Nieuwenhuijsen, ISGlobal, Dr. Aiguader 88,

08003 Barcelona, Spain

Email: mark.nieuwenhuijsen@isglobal.org

OTHER BOOKS PUBLISHED BY THE AUTHOR

Nieuwenhuijsen MJ and Khreis H. (2018) Integrating health into urban and transport planning. Springer. ISBN 978-3-319-74982-2

Nieuwenhuijsen M and Khreis H. (2020) Advances in Transportation and Health1st Edition. Tools, Technologies, Policies, and Developments. Elsevier ISBN: 9780128191361

Khreis H, Nieuwenhuijsen M, Zietsman J and Ramani T (2020) Traffic-Related Air Pollution. Elseviers ISBN: 9780128181225

Acknowledgements

The work presented here was written initially often as posts for blogs. They were only possible because of the wonderful and dedicated people that I work with. I particularly would like to thank our communications department, Pau Rubio, Carolina Pozo, Marta Solano, and Aleix Cabrera, and my personal assistant Mar Ferrer for their input and comments. Furthermore, I would like to thank my group and others working at ISGlobal for providing the inspiration and support to make work so interesting, nice and worthwhile.

Content

FOREWORD

Half the world population lives in cities and this is likely to increase to 70% over the next 20 years. Cities provide jobs, are centres of innovation and wealth creation, but also often are hotspots of air pollution (e.g. particulate matter, NO_2), noise, heat and disease. The high density of buildings and roads can cause so-called urban heat islands, defined as built up areas that are hotter than nearby rural areas. Furthermore, cities often lack accessible green space and physical activity levels of people are below recommended guidelines. They also generate a large proportion of CO_2 emissions, and contribute significantly to the climate crisis. Recent estimates show that 60–80% of final energy use globally is consumed by urban areas and more than 70% of global greenhouse gas emissions are produced within urban areas.

Up to 9 million people die each year because of ambient air pollution levels, 3.2 million because of lack of physical activity and 1.2 million because of traffic accidents. Noise causes more than 1.8 million DALYs a year in Europe alone and heat may cause as much as around 0.4% of premature mortality annually worldwide. A large part of the burden falls on cities as that is where people live and where higher exposure levels are. Population growth, ageing and the climate crisis put a further burden on cities in many aspects, including health

From an urban and transport planning and health view, current urban developments have not been a great success. One of factors that is apparent in all cities is the often large presence of the car that has led to high air pollution and noise levels, CO_2 emissions, heat island effects and lack of physical activity and green space in cities. Public space in many cities is often to a large extent dedicated to motorized traffic (e.g. 60% in a city like Barcelona), even though in many cities it is not the predominant mode of travel (e.g. 25% in a place like Barcelona). Cars either driven or parked (they are parked on average 96% of the time) use space that is now detrimental to health because of e.g. air pollution, noise etc, while it could be used to promote health, if, for example, it was a green space. At times it appears as if that cities are designed for cars rather than for people, while we need cities for people.

The COVID19 pandemic has put renewed focus on cities as hotspots for COVID19 outbreaks due to its connectivity with for example other cities, the high population density and mixing and reliance on public transport. Two of the most effective prevention measures hygiene (including wearing masks) and social distancing have a large effect on the behaviour of citizens, and require a rethink of the urban model and life. Is this the end of the city, or the beginning of the remodelling of the city?

There is good evidence that there is a direct relationship between urban design, how people get around, and how this affects environmental exposure and life style factors and thereby morbidity and mortality. For example, in a city designed for and with large investment in infrastructure for cars, you will get many people using the car. On the other hand, in a city designed for and with investment in infrastructure for active transportation such as cycling, you will get more people cycling. As a result of the pandemic we see many European cities to a model that encourages cycling, partly because people avoid using the public transport system and there is not enough space for everyone to go by car.

In this book I describe the issues and changes in the cities during the pandemic and that, as much as cities may be the problem, they could also be the solution through a transformation in their urban and transport planning practices. It is based on 10 short published posts on blogs between March and September 2020. The bottom line is that the pandemic can be catalyst for change and well planned and managed cities could provide an excellent and efficient habitat for the large human population and could not only be sustainable and liveable, but also healthy. I focus on important interventions, policies and actions that can improve public health, including the need for land use changes, reduce car dependency and move towards public and active transportation, greening of cities, visioning, citizen involvement, collaboration, leadership and investment and systemic approaches.

Mark Nieuwenhuijsen

Barcelona, Spain 20 October 2020

1 COVID-19 AND THE CITY: HOW IS THE PANDEMIC AFFECTING URBAN HEALTH?

The current COVID19 toll stands at 209,839 cases confirmed and 8778 deaths after just a few months and this is likely to increase[1]. The number of cases have overwhelmed health care systems and has led to dramatic actions in e.g. China, Singapore, Japan, Italy, Spain and many other countries. The actions appeared very successful in countries such as China, Singapore and Japan.

Prevention is currently the key through the stay at home programmes, hygiene measures and social distancing, and has led to a large reduction in the number of potential cases that otherwise would overwhelm the health care systems[2,3]

The drastic prevention measures also caused a large reduction in traffic (70-80% or more) and industrial activities, which may have resulted in large reductions in CO_2 emissions and air pollution, up to 20-30% in China[4,5]. A similar reduction is seen in Italy[6], larger in Barcelona (75%)[7] and other places[8].

Reduction in air pollution

Worldwide, every year an estimated 8.8 million people die prematurely of air pollution, which causes an average reduction of 2.9 years in life expectancy[9], 3.2 million die prematurely because of lack of physical activity and 1.35 million because of traffic accidents[10,11]. Furthermore, the climate crisis results in an increasing number of premature deaths[12].

In China, where they are now beyond the peak and for which there is data available, a quick back on the envelope calculation showed that a 25% reduction in air pollution levels for one month may have prevented more than 9000 premature death*, which is higher than the number of deaths due to COVID19 (nearly 4000). And some suggested this may be as high as 77000[13,14]. However, increased indoor air pollution from smoking may have increased the number of premature deaths.

In countries like Italy and Spain, the air pollution levels are much lower to start with than in a China and therefore less premature deaths can be prevented by lower air pollution levels. The number of deaths caused by the COVID19 is likely to be higher than the reduced number caused by lower air pollution levels.

However, lower levels of air pollution may reduce the transmission and fatality rate of COVID19 as was suggested from some SARS research[15,16]

Physical activity

The stay at home programmes may cause a significant reduction in physical activity during that time and lead to an increase in premature mortality. Some preliminary data suggest a reduction in physical activity of 20-30%[17]. Physical activity is very important for physical and mental health, including the immune system. Home exercise may mitigate some of the effects.

There have been calls to allow walking and cycling as part of the stay at home programmes[18]. Although reasonable, the question is how to build this into the stay at home program in a way that it is reasonable and accepted without increasing the risk of contagion. Certainly in the first few weeks, it is advisable not to go outdoors, but for the medium to longer term physical activities outside should be permitted as part of any restrictions.

Car accidents

In China, the reduction in car traffic has led to a large reduction in accidents[19]. In 2016, 256,180 people were killed by car accidents in China[11]. This works out to more than 20,000 fatal accidents per month, which could have been avoided. Reduction in car accidents are likely in other countries, where the stay at home programmes are implemented, but the number of accidents is normally lower, and fewer could be avoided.

Outcomes of economic down turn

The largest impact on public health may come from the economic downturn, including job losses, although the evidence from, for example, the 2007 crisis was quite mixed and it all may depend on the mitigation measures taken[20,21]. The current crisis though looks to be much more severe and may lead to a whole collapse of certain sectors such as aviation, entertainment and tourism, and therefore have much more pronounced consequences on the economy and health. A strong health system needs a strong economy, and what we know now is that a strong economy needs a strong health system.

How should cities respond?

Cities are hotspot of the outbreaks because of e.g. the high population density, close contact of people, high mobility, shared transport and they are gateways, but rural areas have been hit hard too[22]. The advantage though for cities is that they often have better and easier accessible health care systems in place.

Cities are also the solution, as they are centres of innovation, and can be drivers of public health improvement e.g. through better urban and transport planning e.g. by moving away from our car centred approach towards walking and cycling transportation[23,24]. Walking and cycling have the advantage that there is a low risk of contagion, and at the same time it strengthens the lungs and immune system.

The social distancing programs are likely to stay in place for the foreseeable future and we need to prepare our cities for this, for example by providing quickly sufficient and safe infrastructure for walking and cycling to work, which provides opportunities for daily physical activity without causing high air pollution levels, and sufficient and safe public spaces like parks, beaches and other outdoor places, where people can meet and exercise without a high risk of contagion.

In a city like Barcelona 60% of public space is used by cars and this is not the best and most effective way to use public space, if you need a lot of space for people due to social distancing. Innovative approaches on the use of public space are urgently needed.

Social distancing and home containment may lead to loneliness and poor mental health, which are already an issue in cities. How can cities use public space and their services to reduce the impacts? Furthermore, for many of these issues there is an unequal distribution in society with e.g. the more deprived and elderly left behind, and it is important to take measures to mitigate the impacts for these groups and reduce inequalities.

The COVID19 pandemic put public health at the centre of policy making, and shows that drastic actions are possible to reduce the potential number of deaths. Could we have a similar approach to our other large problems that we have such as air pollution, traffic accidents and the climate crisis that cause millions of premature death each year, but without the unwanted side effects on the economy? Can we place prevention rather than treatment at the centre of our policy and decision making?

A wake up call

The COVID19 pandemic is a wakeup call, as our world won´t be the same, and a chance to build better and more sustainable societies and cities. Currently it may give us time to reflect and think about solutions for the long term, while addressing a short term problem. But can we have a permanent paradigm shift, and prevent us falling back into bad old habits?

In the short term we need to focus on the health of colleagues, friends and family and the health care systems. For the medium to long term, we should analyse the data that become available, take a more holistic view of the pandemic, and evaluate, build and implement policies that address health care system requirements, including surveillance, environmental and climate impacts, and governance and can prevent premature death in the short and long term.

Published before in:

https://www.isglobal.org/en/healthisglobal/-/custom-blog-portlet/covid-19-en-las-ciudades-como-esta-afectando-la-pandemia-a-la-salud-urbana-/4735173/0

https://theconversation.com/como-afecta-la-pandemia-a-la-salud-urbana-135704

*There are 2203704 premature preventable deaths due to air pollution each year in China (Lelieveld et al 2020), and assuming a linear relationship between air pollution and deaths, a 1 month reduction of air pollution by 25% and a 5 year exposure period needed to cause premature death, the expected reduction in premature deaths is 9182. It may be an over estimation due to the linearity assumptions and that the estimated reduction may not be for 1 months and equally everywhere.

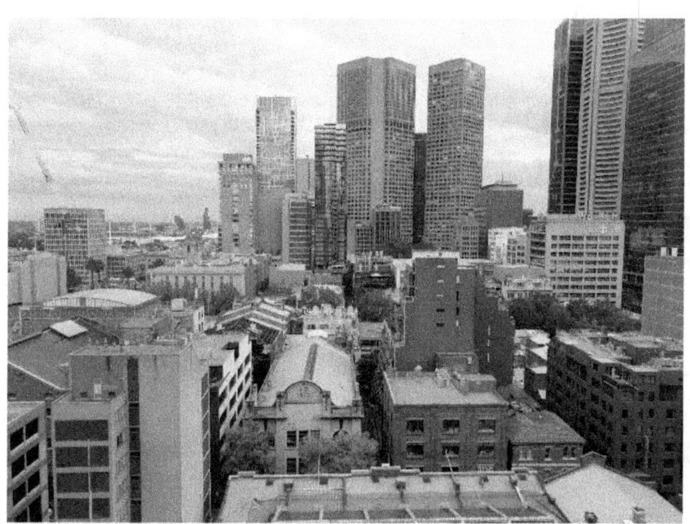

High rises, Melbourne, Australia

2 RECOMMENDATION TO ALLOW PHYSICAL ACTIVITY DURING THE CORONAVIRUS DISEASE PANDEMIC

Overview of Current State

The ubiquitous health benefits of physical activity are scientifically well proven and endorsed by the World Health Organization (WHO)[1,2]. Physical, mental, and social health as well as wellbeing in children, adolescents, adults and seniors are enhanced with regular physical activity. Since March 11th, 2020, when the WHO declared the Coronavirus disease (COVID-19) a pandemic, the majority of countries around the globe employed recommended non-pharmacological interventions (NPIs), including physical distancing and home confinement to decelerate the transmission rate of COVID-19 infections. Spain has implemented one of the strictest NPIs, with complete home confinement, permitting citizens to leave their homes only to access essential services such as grocery shopping, banks, and seeking medical help from pharmacies and hospitals. This level of home confinement has had a drastic effect on individual's physical activity levels. On March 23rd, 2020, after one week of confinement, FitBit (a wearable physical activity tracking service), indicated a decrease of physical activity levels by 38% in Spain[3]. Data up to

April 11th, 2020 provided by Google indicates that physical activity related to recreation and park visits have decreased by 92% and 85%, respectively[4]. As of April 18th, 2020, Spaniards walked 90% less compared to January 13th, 2020[5]. To put this dramatic decrease in physical activity and the subsequent health threat into further perspective: already before the COVID-19 pandemic, only 24% of adolescents, 66% of adults and 68% seniors in Spain met the WHO recommendations for physical activity[6–8]. The health impacts due to this drastic drop in physical activity have not yet been estimated but are anticipated to be broad and dramatic, particularly since deconditioning effects in recreational athletes have been observed to occur within a few weeks already[9].

YouTube videos, and live streaming of physical activity classes have been made freely available online; however, it is unclear how many citizens are truly benefiting from these offers. Inability to access online resources, insufficient knowledge of how to adapt exercise routines safely that are too challenging, limited space and time, missing equipment and motivation are likely key hurdles. Moreover, time outdoors, exposure to vitamin D (the sunshine vitamin), and physical activity ignite a series of health benefits that cannot be achieved to the same extent indoors – ranging from immune function, mood and anxiety, metabolism, heart health, bone health, and overall health and mental well-being. These benefits can be achieved by least 150 minutes of moderate-intensity physical activity throughout the week; with additional health benefits to be gained by increasing the weekly volume of moderate-intensity physical activity to 300 minutes (*i.e.* approximately 30 minutes per day on most days of the week) as per WHO guidelines.[2]

Importance of Access to Outdoor Physical Activity:

Beneficial effects of regular physical activity specifically during the COVID-19 pandemic include:

- Immunological & respiratory health: The coronavirus attacks the lungs and respiratory system by activating inflammatory cascades. Regular physical activity, particularly at low- to moderate intensities, enhances immune competency and has been shown to have an overall anti-inflammatory effect[10,11]. Furthermore, physical activity is important for children's and adult's maintenance of respiratory function[12,13].

- Mental health: Anxiety, fear, and stress are results from the limited current knowledge and uncertainties about the COVID-19 pandemic and the future. Physical activity is a tool to self-manage and release anxiety and stress. It provides an important opportunity for self-care[14,15].

- Metabolic health: The COVID-19 pandemic has undoubtedly changed citizens' dietary behaviours. Increases in high-caloric diets combined with increased alcohol and tobacco consumption are common responses to stressful situations. With no opportunity to engage in physical activity to increase caloric expenditure, weight gain will be unavoidable, resulting in negative health impacts. Physical activity has also been associated with healthier dietary choices, and better sleep quality, which are known to affect body weight.[16,17]

- Cardiovascular health: psychological stress, unbalanced diets, and physical inactivity are key risk factors for cardiovascular disease, all of which have been impacted by the COVID-19 crisis. A reduction in blood pressure, and resting heart rate in response to regular physical activity decreases the risk for myocardial infarctions and strokes, two predominant cardiovascular complications resulting in morbidity or mortality[18].

- Bone health: Due to increases in sedentary time, bone health particularly in children, adolescents and the elderly is at risk. For the growth and maintenance of healthy bones, high forces through impact and shear stress are needed. Body weight bearing physical activities, often completed in activities of daily living such as walking stairs, carrying groceries, running and jumping are often unnoticed factors assisting with bone health[19].

- Social and emotional health: Physical activity helps build and maintain social connectedness. Group exercise programs permit individuals of all ages, professional, and socioeconomic backgrounds to meet and interact, combating the global threat of perceived loneliness[20].

- Other benefits: One of the most repeated recommendations during home confinement is the maintenance of daily routines and structure, especially for mental health. Planning and implementing physical activity routines helps adherence to daily schedules.

Who Can Benefit from Outdoor Physical Activity?

Everyone benefits from outdoor physical activity. However, people with active or recovering COVID-19 infections should consult a physician before resuming exercise. The risk of contracting or transmitting COVID-19 outside appears to be lower compared to indoors[21].

Benefits of outdoor physical activity, particularly in green[22] and blue spaces[23], *i.e.* parks, waterfronts or lakes are numerous, and give particularly those in small apartments without access to a terrace or balcony an opportunity to be physically active. Therefore, access to outdoor physical activity as soon as possible is imperative to prevent greater health threats due to NPIs beyond direct COVID-19 infections.

Physical activity is crucial for children's' organs, immune and other health systems to fully develop, making access to outdoor physical activity essential. Underprivileged individuals such as those in small apartments with no access to gardens, balconies or rooftop terraces should receive priority when deconfinement plans are discussed and implemented. Additionally, individuals with pre-existing health conditions, such as those with medical prescriptions for routine exercise, should be considered.

What Is Needed?

Deconfinement strategies must include urgently opportunities to safely engage in physical activity while permitting citizens to adhere to modified NPIs to minimize COVID-19 infection risk. Measures need to be implemented to permit physical distancing, *i.e.* maintaining a 1.5 meters distance to others at all times, also when engaging in physical activity. For example, walking and cycling are active transport modes that increase physical activity levels, while reducing infection risk when compared to shared, public or private transit. Therefore, considerations should include:

- Provision of space: wider sidewalks and extra cycling lanes, particularly those providing access to green and blue spaces; routes that facilitate active transport to essential services and work need to be urgently implemented. This can be achieved by removing car lanes and parking spaces to make space for bikes on roads while freeing up shared pedestrian and bike space for pedestrian use only.

- Access to large outdoor spaces: Market squares, open areas in parks, roads along waterfronts and lake sides need to be cleared from cars and other obstacles to serve as areas for physical activity with distancing.

- Use of technology to help manage and schedule space use: smartphone applications can be developed to alert citizens to the occupancy of public spaces for exercise near them and suggest alternatives to avoid crowding.

- Tactical Measures to permit physical distancing:

Physical activity should be done alone or with members of the same household and caregivers when necessary.

Generate specific hours for vulnerable citizens when physical activity spaces are exclusively open for them.

Making cycling, jogging, and walking routes one way/one direction use only to generate more capacity.

Extended hours to parks, market squares and physical activity spaces

Marks on the ground indicating 1.5 meters distance to the next.

Arrows on bicycle routes indicating a safe distance to be maintained at all times, similarly to those previously used for drivers

- Access to hand hygiene services: Accessible hand wash and hand sanitizing stations.

- Upregulation of cleaning procedures: public washrooms, handrails at staircases, outdoor gym equipment need to be cleaned more frequently.

Recommendation

Physical activity is essential for good physical, mental, and social health and should be urgently included in the deconfinement strategy. We recommend allowing up to 1 hour of physical activity a day outdoors, with an emphasis that people only exercise by themselves and keep a distance of at least 1.5 meters to others at all times.

Published before in:

https://www.elperiodico.com/es/opinion/20200428
/articulo-mark-nieuwenhuijsen-isglobal-
actividad-fisica-estrategia-desconfinamiento-
7943482

Monica Ubalde, Sarah Koch and Carolyn Daher contributed to this chapter

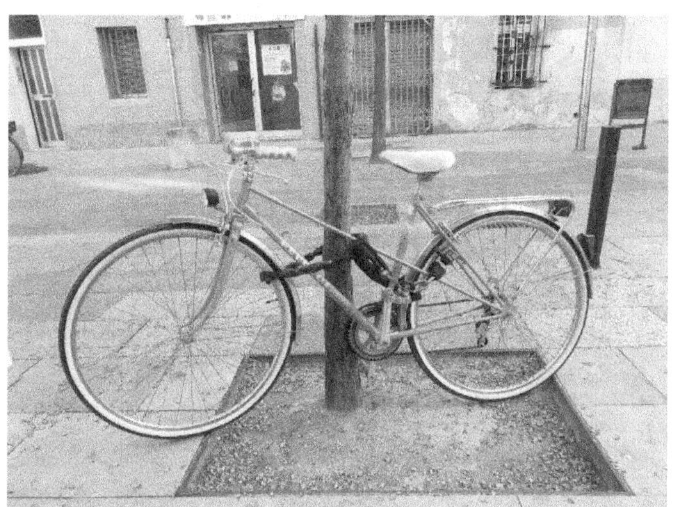

Parked bike, Barcelona, Spain

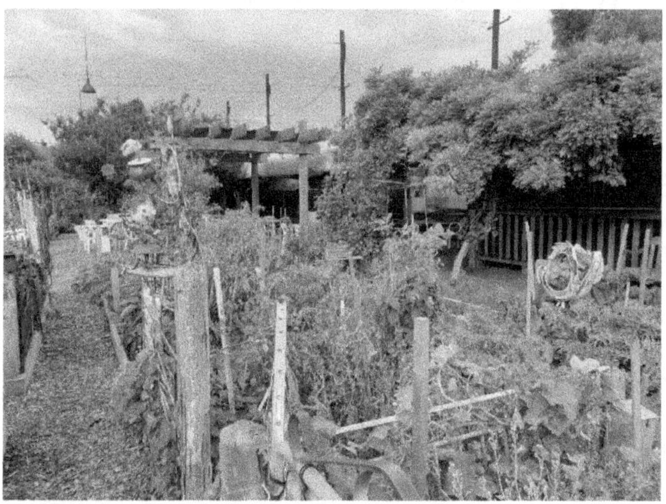

Urban garden, Melbourne, Australia

3 COULD THE COVID19 CRISIS BE THE OPPORTUNITY TO MAKE CITIES CARBON NEUTRAL, LIVEABLE AND HEALTHY

It may be the time to turn a tragic emergency into a catalyst for change.

COVID-19 has hit the entire society hard. A collateral victim of the current pandemic may be all the actions addressed to manage the climate crisis. This is evidenced by, for example, COP26 postponement. Furthermore, the ambitious European green deal funding priorities may be overtaken by those for the COVID-19 pandemic. The short-term emergency threatening the necessary long-term requirements is nothing new but, does it need to be this way? Can't we create a win-win scenario?

The COVID19 pandemic requires a large financial stimulus package which creates opportunities for change, and possibly for the better. We cannot simply continue the way we did, and therefore any stimulus packages should be holistic and not only include requirements and indicators for the economy, but also for equity, sustainability, liveability and health. The money can only be spent once, and we therefore might as well do it in the way that will save more lives in the long term, and create a more just, sustainable and liveable society.

According to data from the United Nations, 55% of the world's population lives in urban areas, a proportion that is expected to increase to 68% by 2050. Suboptimal urban and transport planning in cities has led them to be hotspots of air pollution and noise, heat island effects and lack of green space. What are the effects of these conditions?

Outdoor air pollution alone kills 9 million people a year- a number that could be significantly reduced as the current COVID-19 pandemic has shown. A recent health impact assessment study in Barcelona found that around 20% of premature mortality was due to factors related to suboptimal urban and transport planning. Cities are also large emitters of CO_2, one of the main factors behind the climate crisis.

Cities might be the problem, but also the solution as they are centres of innovation and wealth creation and tend to be more responsive and agile in their governance. As part of any stimulus package, cities could and should take measures to become carbon neutral, more liveable and healthier by changing their current urban and transport planning practices. Some measures to be taken are as follows[1]:

Land use changes

To address this, several issues must be considered. First of all, higher population and development density lead often to shorter travel distances because destinations become closer to origins. It is also important to have diversity, characterised by a mix of homes, shops, schools, and work places in an area. And, finally, a better design that includes connectivity and infrastructure for cycling and walking should be aimed for. All of which lead to more walking, cycling and public transport use and reduce car use.

The actual design, use of space and traffic, air quality and green space management are important. For example, in Barcelona a new urban model is proposed, the so-called Superblock (SuperIlles in Catalan) that aims to recover public space for people and thereby reduce car use, air pollution, noise and temperature levels and increase green space and physical activity. It could prevent almost 700 deaths annually.

Reduce car dependency and move towards public and active transportation

Currently there are around 1 billion cars in the world and this number is likely to rise: at times it looks like cities are made for cars instead of for people. Electric and autonomous cars have been suggested as solutions to air pollution and noise, but they do not address the lack of physical activity and still use a lot of public space that could be used better.

A large number of car trips (as high as 50%) are less than 5 kilometers long and these could easily be replaced by other modes of transport such as cycling. Cycling has many advantages as it reduces e.g. premature mortality, it combines transport with the gym (many people don't have time to go to the gym), it does not cause air and noise pollution, it emits zero

CO_2, it uses much less space than the car and cyclists tend to be happier than other transport users.

A recent study in 167 cities in Europe found that more than 10.000 premature deaths could be avoided annually if the bicycle share mode raised 25% in these cities. Cycling has important prerequisites, though, such as the availability of safe cycling infrastructure including segregated cycling lanes.

Greening of cities

Greening cities has obvious benefits, such as air pollution, heat and noise mitigation, carbon sequestration and offsetting carbon emissions. Behind all these effects, there are plenty of health benefits: longer life expectancy, fewer mental health problems, better cognitive functioning, better mood and healthier babies.

As an example, a recent study estimated that more than 400 premature deaths overall, including more than 200 deaths in lower SES areas, could be prevented annually in Philadelphia, if the city is able to meet its goal of increasing tree canopy from its current 20% to up to 30%.

Visioning

What may be lacking in many cities is probably a vision of what is a sustainable, liveable and healthy city, and how to put this vision into standard operating procedures. There is no cook book out there on what are the ingredients of such a city and how to prepare it. But it is urgently needed.

A number of cities have a vision to become car free e.g. Hamburg envisages to be car free by 2034. The main driver is climate action, but it may have also many benefits for liveability and health. A good example of a car free neighbourhood is Vauban in Freiburg.

Citizen involvement

There is also a need to involve more the citizens. As where in the past many larger developments were top down, nowadays there is a large need to involve the community and citizens in any urban and transport planning development, and have a bottom up approach.

An interesting and novel approach has been taken by the Ringland project in Antwerp, Belgium. This initiative is a 6-billion-euro investment, which proposes a large-scale sustainable urban development focusing on a complete redesign of the highway system in the city of Antwerp. The research underlying this complex infrastructure project has been entirely organized by local citizens in bottom-up fashion. Detailed research studies, executed by external academics, were financed through crowdfunding and subsequently presented to the government.

Collaboration, leadership and investment

There is a large need for collaboration to improve current cities. This requires collaboration between urban and transport planners, architects, the education section and health professionals, to name a few. Good leadership and the right investment is essential and mayors and their teams need to take the lead and direct investments that benefit these different aspects in cities. Unfortunately, too often we find a lack of leadership and focus and too many silos in cities.

There are some bright spots though. Cities have taken the lead in sustainability and climate crisis and are more networked than ever. They have enhanced their capabilities by working together, sharing experiences and forging public–private partnerships across health, governance, democracy, infrastructure and security. Formal networks include C40 Cities Climate Leadership Group, the Rockefeller Foundation's 100 Resilient Cities, United Cities and Local Governments (UCLG), ICLEI Local Governments for Sustainability and the World Health Organization's (WHO) Healthy Cities.

Systemic approaches

Cities are complex systems and to address their challenges we need system approaches taking into many different factors. It requires an effort to install this type of thinking and action that ticks many boxes, but also take into account feedback loops. It is important that we have a more holistic approach to our cities, addressing health, livability, sustainability, climate change and equity simultaneously.

Equity

Finally, we know that environmental exposures and lifestyle factors, and thereby health, are often not equally distributed through cities. We see gradients of life expectancy in cities, and part of them can be explained by these different factors. In any of the proposed measures equity should be fully considered.

In conclusion

Better urban and transport planning can lead to carbon neutral, more liveable and healthier cities. The current COVID19 pandemic requires a rethink of our cities as, for example, social distancing measures are likely to stay in place. Now may be the time to turn a tragic emergency into a great catalyst for change for the better.

Published before in:
https://sites.google.com/view/uhwb/publications/featured-publications

https://www.elperiodico.com/es/opinion/20200514/covid-cambio-modelo-urbano-articulo-mark-nieuwenhuijsen-7962252

https://theconversation.com/ensenanzas-del-coronavirus-8-medidas-para-hacer-ciudades-mas-habitables-y-saludables-136807

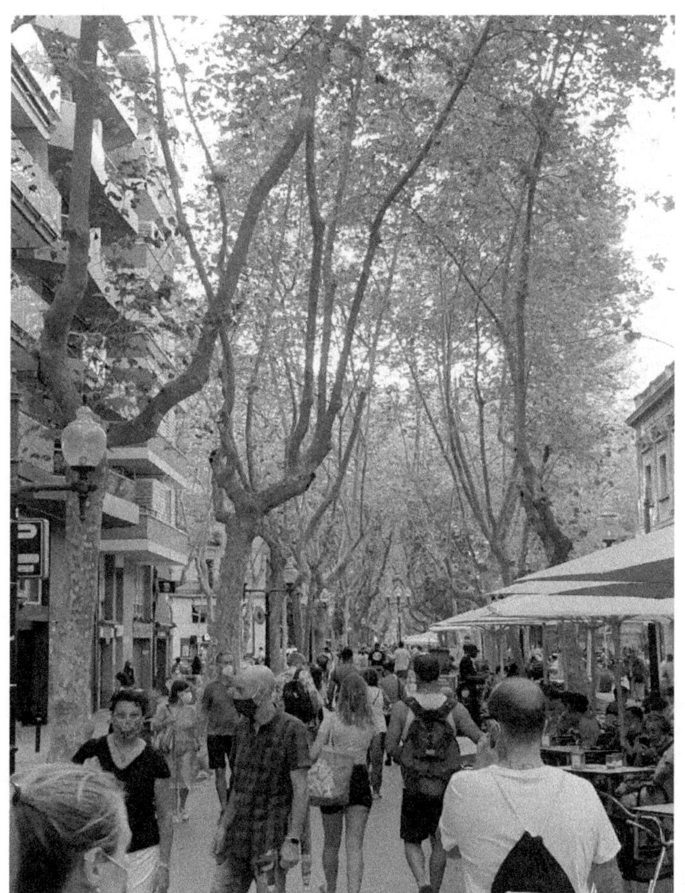

Rambla de Poblenou, Barcelona, Spain

4 AFTER THE LOCKDOWN, HOW ARE WE GOING COMMUTE TO WORK; BY CAR OR BY BICYCLE?

There is a large need for safe, sustainable and healthy mobility

Sooner or later we will go back to work and sooner or later we are going to need to make a decision: how are we going to commute? The answer to this question has health implications, not only at individual level, but also at community level. Safety is a factor of concern, but there are others.

Some of the most effective measures to reduce the transmission of COVID19 are the physical distancing measures (1.5 metres distance) and hygiene (e.g. hand washing) and they are likely to stay in place for the rest of the year and we need to observe them while commuting.

During the lockdown we have seen large reductions in air pollution and noise levels in cities due to a large reduction in motorized traffic, but also unfortunately a reduction in physical activity and an increase in poor mental health. The lower levels of air pollution and noise are being welcomed by many citizens. Physical activity is essential for good mental and physical health.

Public transport was an important mode of transport before the COVID19 pandemic, but has suffered a loss of confidence because of the perceived higher risk of transmission of COVID19. Many measures need to be taken to bring back confidence including the prevention of overcrowding as not return to public transport for sardines. Walking is a popular and good alternative, but generally only possible for short distances (up to a few kilometres).

So the car appears to be a good option to get around, but is it?

The car is the perfect physical distance measure, provides comfort and is generally the fastest transport mode to get somewhere, partly due to the large investments in infrastructure needed for it like roads and parking[1]. However, it is also expensive, it is a sedentary activity that reduces overall physical activity and it needs a lot of public space that can be used in better ways. In a city like Barcelona, 60% of public space is taken up by the car.

Also, if everyone would want to use the car, there will be tremendous congestion problems in many places. Furthermore, the car makes a large contribution to air pollution, noise and carbon emissions in cities (and there are similar concerns for motorbikes)[1]

Outdoor air pollution alone kills 9 million people a year- and levels of air pollution could be significantly reduced as the current COVID-19 pandemic has shown. A recent health impact assessment study in Barcelona found that around 20% of premature mortality was due to factors related to suboptimal urban and transport planning[2]. Cities are also large emitters of CO_2, one of the main factors behind the climate crisis.

Is cycling the solution?

A large number of car trips are less than 5 kilometers (as high as 50%) and these could easily be replaced by other more sustainable and healthier modes of transport such as cycling. Cycling has many benefits as it increases physical activity and reduces e.g. premature mortality, it combines transport with the gym (many people don't have time to go to the gym), it does not cause air and noise pollution, it emits zero CO2 (although some through the manufacturing and what the rider eats), it uses much less space than the car and cyclists tend to be happier than other transport users[3].

Also, as many people have gained weight during confinement, the bicycle is an excellent way to lose weight. A number of studies have shown that cyclists weigh less than car drivers, and that also car drivers who switch to cycling lose weight[4].

Electric bikes have become more popular over the past few years as the prices have come down. Electric bikes allow older people to cycle and also is good for cycling in hilly areas as they require less effort. But they still provide physical activity[5]. In the Netherland and Belgium electric bikes have become popular for long distance commuting with distances up to 30 kilometers.

And what do driving a car and cycling do to our wallet?

The COVID19 pandemic is hitting us hard economically. Cost benefit analyses show that costs of cycling are general much lower than car use; for example, the cost of car driving is more than six times higher (Euro 0.50/km) than cycling (Euro 0.08/km) in Copenhagen[6].

What do we need to do to get people cycling?

What deters many people from cycling is safety. Accidents rates for cyclists are still considerably higher than for example for cars (although accident rates for motor bikes are even worse). Therefore, an important prerequisite for cycling though is e.g. the availability of safe cycling infrastructure, including segregated cycling lanes. Cities urgently need to create safe cycling networks throughout the city, or free up some streets altogether for only cycling and walking. Putting a safe segregated cycling lane in each street could save 250 premature deaths annually in a city like Barcelona[7]. Also, reducing car speeds to maximum of 30 kilometers per hour will help to reduce accidents in the remaining roads.

A great opportunity to be taken

The COVID19 pandemic is a great opportunity to make changes that allow for more sustainable, liveable and healthy cities, but we need to make the changes rapidly[8]. Cycling is a great sustainable and healthy alternative for many car trips, but safe cycling networks are urgently needed not only within cities, but also between cities, town and villages to allow for sustainable and healthy mobility that will have long term benefits.

Published before in:

https://www.isglobal.org/en/healthisglobal/-/custom-blog-portlet/tras-el-confinamiento-como-iremos-a-trabajar-en-coche-o-en-bici-/4735173/0

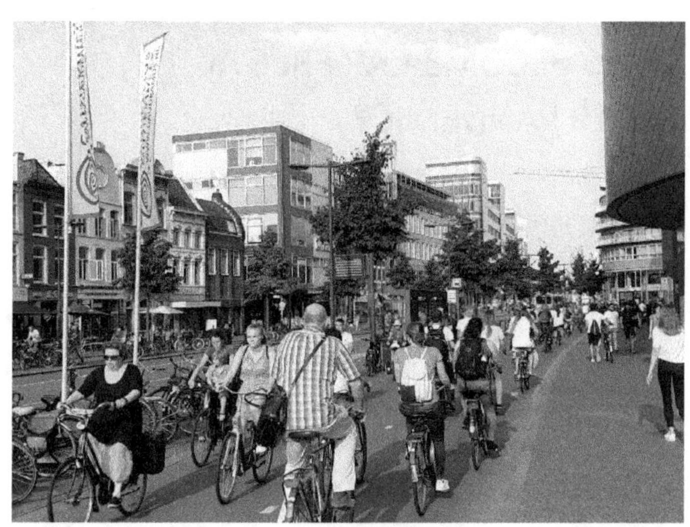

Cycling, Utrecht, the Netherlands

5 CAN CITIES BECOME CAR FREE AFTER THE COVID19 PANDEMIC?

Cities and COVID19

The COVID19 pandemic has hit society and cities hard[1]. Measures like physical distancing (1.5 meter distance) and good hygiene (i.e. washing) are effective and are likely to stay in place for the foreseeable future. Many cities are rethinking their transport systems and are making changes.

Many cities including Barcelona, London, Madrid, Milan and Paris are now extending public space to pedestrians and cyclist to further encourage these modes of transport, and to allow for sufficient distance between people. This often comes at the expense of space used by cars. Before the COVID19 pandemic, in a city like Barcelona, 60% of public space was taken up by the car[2].

By reducing the road space for cars, and thereby reducing the use of cars, an interesting question arises; can these cities go car free?

During the lockdown we have seen large reductions in motorized traffic that caused large reductions in air pollution and noise levels in cities. The lower levels of air pollution and noise were being welcomed by many citizens. Fresher air could be breathed in and birds could be heard singing again.

Outdoor air pollution alone kills 9 million people a year- and levels of air pollution could be significantly reduced as the COVID-19 pandemic has shown. A recent health impact assessment study in Barcelona found that around 20% of premature mortality was due to factors related to suboptimal urban and transport planning. Cities are also large emitters of CO_2, one of the main factors behind the climate crisis.

Going car free

A number of cities have a vision to become car free e.g. Hamburg envisages to be car free by 2034[3]. The main driver is climate action. Car free cities can also have a considerable benefit on public health through potential reduction in air pollution, noise, and heat island effects and increase in physical activity and green space and thereby improving health[3].

Many cities in Europe like Helsinki, Madrid and Oslo have tried to pedestrianize the city centre or some neighbourhood. A nice example of a fairly large car free neighbourhood with sustainable housing is Vauban in Freiburg[3]. No cars are allowed in the neighbourhood and there are good transport links to the centre of the city e.g. by tram[4].

What could be consider car free?

Here I consider a car free city as a city without private cars, but one that may still have a small number of e.g. buses, lorries, taxis, and emergency vehicles as necessary to move goods and people, when essential.

The characteristics are that by far the largest mode share is taken by public and active transport and that these are also the modes at the top of the hierarchy for transport planning and engineering. Furthermore, the motor vehicles remaining on the roads should be as sustainable and healthy as possible - e.g. by being electric, having speed restrictions as well as other restrictions in terms of time and areas of the city they can be.

The transport mode share of private cars in many cities is often relatively low as active and public transportation account for the bulk of mode share.   It also suggests that becoming car free is not so far away after all.

Can we retrofit cities and change mode share?

Compact cities like many European type cities may be easier to refit to car free cities than sprawled cities like American or Australian type cities[5]. The main challenges will be how to change existing infrastructure that was mainly designed for cars to infrastructure for active and public transport, and how to change people´s perceptions, attitudes and behaviors. Some cities have initiated strategies to create largely car free areas like the Super blocks in Barcelona. A recent health impact assessment study found that nearly 700 premature deaths could be prevented if all 502 Superblocks would be implemented[6].

A large number of car trips are less than 7 kilometers (as high as half) and these could easily be replaced by other more sustainable and healthier modes of transport such as cycling[7]. Cycling has many benefits as it increases physical activity and reduces e.g. premature mortality, it combines transport with the gym (many people don't have time to go to the gym), it does not cause air and noise pollution, it emits near zero CO_2, it uses much less space than the car and cyclists tend to be happier than other transport users[8].

What is needed to go car free?

There are a number of important factors to address when aiming to go car free and they include:

- Political vision and leadership
- Mobility to accessibility paradigm shift
- Alternative convenient and quality transport means
- Dedicated funding
- Media strategy and public involvement and acceptability
- Intensive data collection and analysis
- Evaluation of current status, alternative scenarios, and post-evaluation of policies impacts
- Stakeholders involvements and support
- Detailed plan aligned with other high-level objectives and strategies

(After Nieuwenhuijsen et al 2019)[9]

Can cities go car free?

Given the relatively small transport mode share of cars in many cities, they are moving towards going car free, but unfortunately the streets are still dominated by cars. This is partly because even though the mode share is relatively small, there are still have hundreds of thousands of cars on the road, and because each car takes up of a lot of space. Cities spend still too much money on keeping car drivers happy, and too little on other road users. Therefore, a more concerted effort is needed to push for a reduction in car use and create car free streets and neighbourhoods in a move towards a car free city. Also any new urban development should be car free and provide good alternatives. Supporting more the local economy and creating a 15 minute city like in Paris with mixed land use are essential[10].

What holds us back from going car free?

Decades of planning and investments in car infrastructure attracted cars to the cities and it will take decades to overturn this. Large car-oriented infrastructures continue to dominate with relatively small proportions of the budget allocated to and little work done for quality active and public transport provision across most regions. There is an urgent need to rebalance and provide better and safer infrastructures and policy support for active and public transport modes. For many the car is still a status symbol and the fastest, easiest and most comfortable way to get around, and negative impacts such as air pollution, noise, heat island effects and

CO2 emissions are too easily ignored. Further, retail interest and the car interest groups may be some of the biggest barriers, but the concerns are often unfounded.

A car free city would provide a catalyst for better town planning by removing the need to facilitate car mobility and ensuring that urban areas are planned around people, functionality and better built environments instead.

Published as:

https://www.urbanet.info/car-free-cities-after-pandemic/

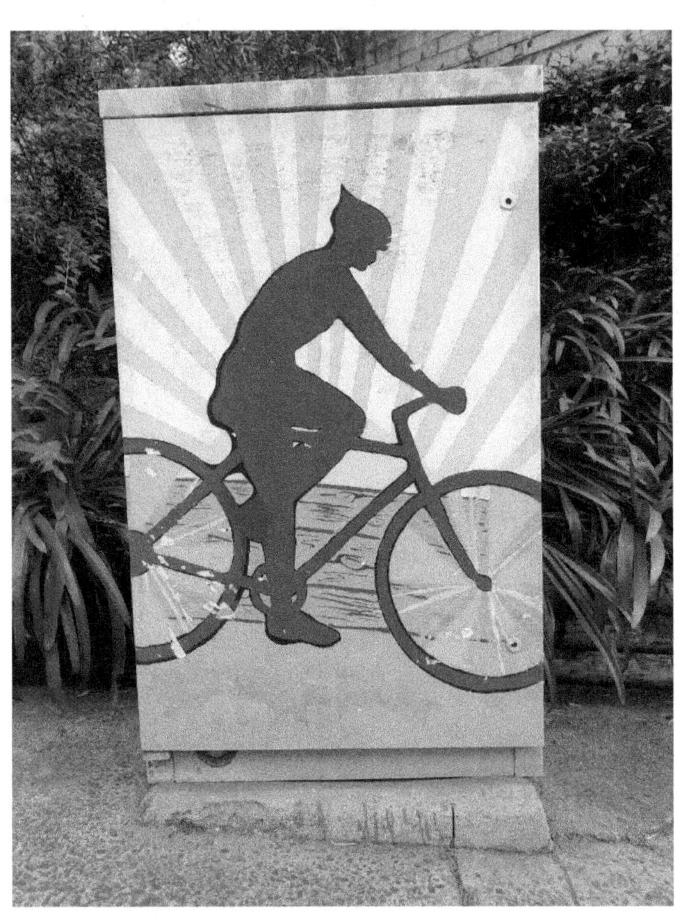

Painted bicycle, Sydney Australia,

6 CAN SPANISH CITIES LIKE BILBAO, BARCELONA, MADRID, SEVILLE AND VALENCIA BECOME CAR FREE?

Cities and COVID19

The COVID19 pandemic has hit society and cities hard[1]. Some of the strictest home confinement measures were applied in Spain. Measures like physical distancing (1.5 meter distance) and good hygiene (i.e. washing) are effective and are likely to stay in place for the foreseeable future. Cities are rethinking their transport systems and are making changes.

Many cities including Barcelona and Madrid are now extending public space to pedestrians and cyclist to further encourage these modes of transport, and to allow for sufficient distance between people. This often comes at the expense of space used by cars. Before the COVID19 pandemic, in a city like Barcelona, 60% of public space was taken up by the car[2].

By reducing the road space for cars, and thereby reducing the use of cars, an interesting question arises; can these cities go car free?

During the lockdown we have seen large reductions in motorized traffic that caused large reductions in air pollution and noise levels in cities. The lower levels of air pollution and noise were being welcomed by many citizens. Fresher air could be breathed in and birds could be heard singing again.

Outdoor air pollution alone kills 9 million people a year- and levels of air pollution could be significantly reduced as the COVID-19 pandemic has shown. A recent health impact assessment study in Barcelona found that around 20% of premature mortality was due to factors related to suboptimal urban and transport planning. Cities are also large emitters of CO_2, one of the main factors behind the climate crisis.

Going car free

A number of cities have a vision to become car free e.g. Hamburg envisages to be car free by 2034[3]. The main driver is climate action. Car free cities can also have a considerable benefit on public health through potential reduction in air pollution, noise, and heat island effects and increase in physical activity and green space and thereby improving health[3].

Many cities in Europe like Helsinki and Oslo have tried to pedestrianize the city centre or some neighbourhood. A nice example of a fairly large car free neighbourhood with sustainable housing is Vauban in Freiburg[3]. No cars are allowed in the neighbourhood and there are good transport links to the centre of the city e.g. by tram[4].

Pontevedra is a small car-free city in Spain. Cars are banned from Pontevedra's city center, creating a model for a pedestrian-friendly future. In the car-free zone, CO2 emissions have been cut significantly and walkers are free to roam.

What could be consider car free?

Here we consider a car free city as a city without private cars, but one that may still have a small number of e.g. buses, lorries, taxis, and emergency vehicles as necessary to move goods and people, when essential. The characteristics are that by far the largest mode share is taken by public and active transport and that these are also the modes at the top of the hierarchy for transport planning and engineering. Furthermore, the motor vehicles remaining on the roads should be as sustainable and healthy as possible - e.g. by being electric, having speed restrictions as well as other restrictions in terms of time and areas of the city they can be.

The current transport mode share of private transport in Bilbao, Barcelona, Madrid, Seville and Valencia varies from 20% to 43%, suggesting that a lower mode share by car is possible in many of the cities (Table 1). It also suggests that becoming car free is not so far away.

Table 1 Modeshare (%) in Spanish cities (2018)

	Active modes	Public transport	Private transport	Others
Barcelona[1]	46,4	33,3	20,3	0.0
Madrid[2]	40.0	35.0	20.0	5.0
Sevilla[3]	32.3	20.1	43.4	4.2
Bilbao[4]	54.5	22.3	23.2	0.0
Valencia[5]	38.5	22.5	37.3	1.7

Table prepared by Guillem Vich, ISGlobal

Can we retrofit cities and change mode share?

Compact cities like Spanish cities may be easier to refit to car free cities than sprawled cities[5]. The main challenges will be how to change existing infrastructure that was mainly designed for cars to infrastructure for active and public transport, and how to change people´s perceptions, attitudes and behaviors. Some cities have initiated strategies to create car free spaces like the Super blocks in Barcelona. A recent health impact assessment study found that nearly 700 premature deaths could be prevented if all 502 Superblocks would be implemented[6]. In Madrid, the Madrid central was initiated, but lost impact with a change in local governance.

A large number of car trips are less than 7 kilometers (as high as half) and these could easily be replaced by other more sustainable and healthier modes of transport such as cycling[7]. Cycling has many benefits as it increases physical activity and reduces e.g. premature mortality, it combines transport with the gym (many people don't have time to go to the gym), it does not cause air and noise pollution, it emits near zero CO2, it uses much less space than the car and cyclists tend to be happier than other transport users[8].

What is needed to go car free?

There are a number of important factors to address when aiming to go car free and they include:

- Political vision and leadership
- Mobility to accessibility paradigm shift
- Alternative convenient and quality transport means
- Dedicated funding
- Media strategy and public involvement and acceptability
- Intensive data collection and analysis
- Evaluation of current status, alternative scenarios, and post-evaluation of policies impacts
- Stakeholders involvements and support
- Detailed plan aligned with other high-level objectives and strategies

(After Nieuwenhuijsen et al 2019)[9]

Can Spanish cities go car free?

Given the relatively small transport mode share of cars, Spanish cities (table 1) are moving towards going car free, but unfortunately the streets are still dominated by cars. This is partly because even though the mode share is relatively small, there are still have hundreds of thousands of cars on the road, and because each car takes up of a lot of space. Cities spend still too much money on keeping car drivers happy, and too little on other road users. Therefore, a more concerted effort is needed to push for a reduction in car use and create car free streets and neighbourhoods in a move towards a car free city. Also any new urban development should be car free and provide good alternatives. Supporting more the local economy and creating a 15-minute city with mixed land use are essential[10].

What holds us back from going car free?

Decades of planning and investments in car infrastructure attracted cars to the cities and it will take decades to overturn this. Large car-oriented infrastructures continue to dominate with relatively small proportions of the budget allocated to and little work done for quality active and public transport provision across most regions. There is an urgent need to rebalance and provide better and safer infrastructures and policy support for active and public transport modes. For many the car is still a status symbol and the fastest, easiest and most comfortable way to get around, and negative impacts such as air pollution, noise, heat island effects and CO_2 emissions are too easily ignored. Further, retail interest and the car interest groups may be some of the biggest barriers, but the ·concerns are often unfounded.

A car free city would provide a catalyst for better town planning by removing the need to facilitate car mobility and ensuring that urban areas are planned around people, functionality and better built environments instead.

Published before in:

https://theconversation.com/pueden-las-ciudades-espanolas-prescindir-del-coche-139482

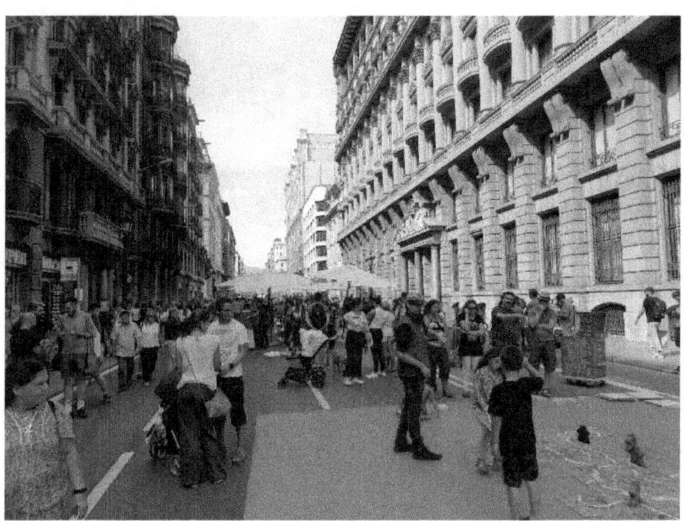

Car free day, Via Laietana, Barcelona, Spain

7 WHY CITIES NEED GREEN SPACE MORE THAN EVER

As a result of the COVID10 pandemic and subsequent lockdown, we have seen an increase in stress, poor mental health, domestic violence and calls for divorce. The confinement together with the economic downturn, resulting in many lay-offs, are some of the obvious causes.

Numerous studies have shown that the presence of greenness and visits to green space can reduce stress and improve restoration of the brain, and thereby improve mental health[1]. Green space is essential for good physical and mental health.

During the lockdown in Catalonia, there was 90% reduction in green space visits as a result of the restrictions[2], reducing people´s resilience

But unfortunately in cities we see often too little green space such as parks, forest or trees in roads. The World Health Organisation recommends that everyone has a green space of at least 0.5 hectare within 300 metres of their house[3], but many people don't, particularly in poorer areas.

Greening cities has many health benefits including longer life expectancy, fewer mental health problems, better cognitive functioning, better mood and healthier babies[4]. It also mitigates air pollution, heat and noise levels. It adds to CO2 sequestration and therefore helps in our fight again the climate crisis. And green space can improve ecosystems and increase biodiversity in cities, particularly through well designed green infrastructure through the city[5].

A recent study showed that children who went to a school with more greenspace had a considerably better cognitive functioning than those who went to a school with less greenspace[6], while another study found that early child hood exposure to green space leads to fewer mental health problems in adult life[7]

Multiple studies have found that green space reduces premature mortality, and increasing tree canopy from 20% to 30% in a city like Philadelphia could avoid more than 400 premature deaths annually[8]. Particularly poorer neighbourhoods would benefit.

Replacing roads and car parking with green environments can be one way forward to change an environment from detrimental to beneficial for sustainability, liveable and health[9]. Before the COVID19 pandemic, in a city like Barcelona, 60% of public space was taken up by infrastructure for the car[10]. New urban models like the Barcelona Superblocks could increase green space and thereby improving health[11].

But it is not only green space that has many benefits, also bluespace like rivers, lakes and the sea, as they could provide space for restoration[12].

Some of the most effective measures to reduce the transmission of COVID19 are physical distancing measures (1.5 metres distance), hygiene (e.g. hand washing) and being outdoors as the transmission risk of COVID19 is very low compared to indoors.

More than ever there is a need for more and larger outdoor natural public spaces such as parks, forests, road trees, rivers, lakes and seas provide great public spaces, as they not only reduce the transmission risk of COVID19, but also reduce stress and improve restoration. They are a great resource for people and society and an increased effort should be made to maintain and improve them to improve our mental health.

Published before in

https://www.isglobal.org/en/healthisglobal/-/custom-blog-portlet/-por-que-las-ciudades-necesitan-espacios-verdes-mas-que-nunca-/4735173/0

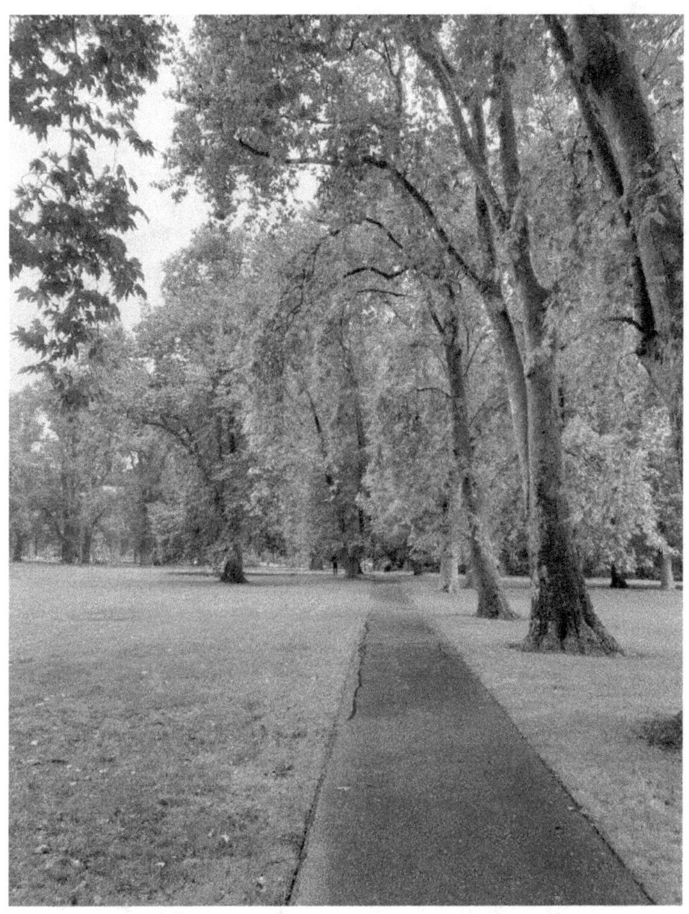

Fitzroy gardens, Melbourne, Australia

8 BUILDING RESILIENCE TO COVID19

The COVID19 pandemic is still ongoing, with no end in sight. Prevention measures such as hand washing, social distancing and wearing masks, particularly in enclosed public space are essential, but not always easy to maintain in the long term. Transmissions appear to be more often taking place during private social events such as dinners, weddings and birthdays parties. The opening of bars and nightclubs also has led to some to some outbreaks, and they are being closed again.

Many people pin their hope on a vaccine to counter the virus, but even though that many vaccines are being developed, it may take a long time before they are actually on the market and people get vaccinated. In the meanwhile, we need to focus more on prevention and building up resilience. In people, resilience is the ability to withstand adversity and bounce back from difficult life events. Community resilience is the sustained ability of a community to use the available resources (e.g. urban planning, transportation, food etc) to respond to, withstand and recover from adverse events. How do we build resilience?

Personal resilience

Smoking, obesity and lack of physical activity have all been linked with either higher transmission risk and/or the severity of the COVID19[1]. Too many people still smoke, are overweight and/or lack physical activity.

To increase resilience it is important to give up smoking, keep your weight within a healthy range (body mass index between 18.5 and 24.9) and get enough physical activity (at least 150 minutes of moderate or vigorous physical activity per week).

We know that physical is important to keep the immune system functioning well and a healthy immune system is important to prevent against and in the fight against COVID19[2,3].

Visiting parks, nature and other green space can reduce stress and improve restoration of the brain, and thereby improve mental health and build resilience[4]. Green space is essential for good physical and mental health. Also, outdoors the transmission risk of COVID-19 is very low compared to indoors.

Finally, healthy eating habits with for example sufficient vegetables and fruit consumption is important for a good immune system and general[5]. The Immune system is built on beneficial live bacteria that lives in the gut (built from fiber-rich foods) which protect the human body from disease. Plant-based foods improve the gut microbiome and therefore the immune system[6]

Community resilience

A good, efficient and well-functioning health care system is essential, particular a good contact tracing system. Contact tracing is the process of identifying, assessing, and managing people who have been exposed to a disease to prevent onward transmission. When systematically applied, contact tracing will break the chains of transmission of an infectious disease and is thus an essential public health tool for controlling infectious disease outbreaks[7].

One of the important prevention measures is social distancing (1.5 meter or so). Therefore, we need sufficient public space in cities for people to be able to keep distance, while walking or cycling particularly. Much of the public space in cities is often used by car, even though that often it is not the main mode of transport (walking is).

Therefore, we should create more space for walking and cycling, and increase physical activity. Many European cities are already doing this, but more efforts are needed[8]. New urban design concepts such as Superblocks (Barcelona), 15-minute city (Paris) and Car free cities (Hamburg) should be promoted and the motorised traffic speed on the remaining roads reduced to 30 km/hrs to create more and safer public space[9].

Air pollution increase the risk of COVID19 infection and disease, possibly because it increases susceptibility[10]. Cities are hotspots of air pollution, but air pollution levels can be reduced as we have seen during the recent lockdowns. Stronger efforts should be made to reduce current air pollution levels to reduce the risk of COVID19 for example by severely reducing and electrifying motorized traffic and using cleaner household fuels from renewable resources.

People spend up to 90% of their time in time insight, and in the indoor environment, including at home, there is a much greater transmission risk than outside. Sufficient ventilation can reduce the risk of transmissions significantly and a well-engineered ventilation system and/or opening windows is essential[11].

Comorbidity

Not smoking, a healthy weight, physical activity, green space visits, healthy diet and a reduction in air pollution are not only important to withstand the COVID19 virus, but are also important to reduce diseases in general like cardiovascular and respiratory disease, diabetes, cancer and Alzheimer´s disease and reduce the risk of premature mortality. Many people died of COVID19 because they had an already existing disease, and therefore reducing disease rates will reduce COVID19 related mortality.

In conclusion

The resilience measures may not fully eliminate COVID19, but may reduce the risk of transmission and disease. Personal and community level resilience go hand in hand, and our communities determine how we behave. A stronger effort is needed to build sustainable, liveable and resilient cities that lead to more resilient and healthy people. These measures would result in long term impacts on our cities and people.

First published in: https://www.isglobal.org/en/healthisglobal/-/custom-blog-portlet/construyendo-resiliencia-frente-a-la-covid-19/4735173/0

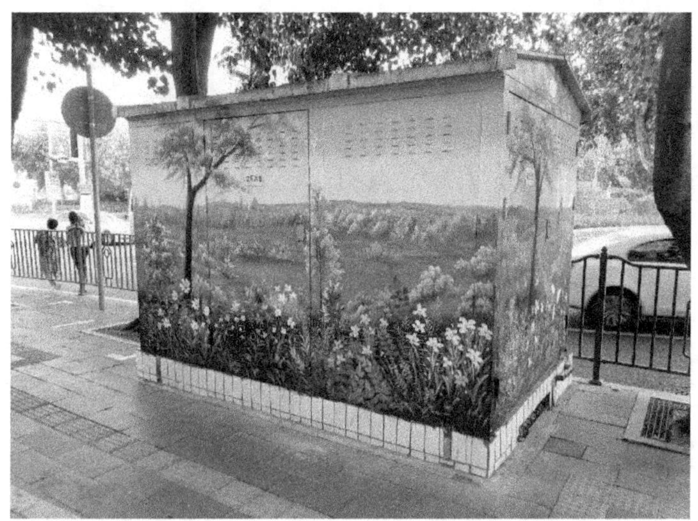

Painted green space, Xiamen, China

9 RADICAL CHANGES IN URBAN AND TRANSPORT PLANNING ARE NEEDED FOR A HEALTHIER BARCELONA; THE NEW PLAN CERDÀ FOR 21ST CENTURY.

Introduction

The COVID19 pandemic has hit Barcelona very hard, with the most noticeable visible impacts the lack of tourists, shop closures, underused public transport and the use of masks. During the severe lockdown, car and motor bike traffic fell dramatically resulting in a drop of air pollution and noise levels. Before the pandemic Barcelona had some of the highest traffic density and air pollution and noise levels in Europe, and suboptimal urban and transport planning has led to an estimated 3000 premature deaths per year[1]

Barcelona is a compact city with some of the highest population and traffic densities in Europe, and it forms part of a large metropolitan area. Even though only around 1 out of 4 trips in Barcelona is taking by car, car traffic dominates the city because of its large demand for space and infrastructure. Furthermore, there is a lack of green space in the city with only a few parks.

The city council is trying to address these issue and try to reduce space for cars and increase space for pedestrians and cyclists e.g. creating so called Superblocks and by increasing dramatically cycling lanes, but the progress is slow[2]. A large part of the problem is traffic coming from the metropolitan area with around 500,000 cars entering and leaving Barcelona city every day.

Furthermore, there are other underlying trends such as the online buying of products that requires delivery of millions of packages per year and death of local shops. During the pandemic online buying has doubled to around an estimated 20% of products sold online now. Also, because of various reasons Barcelona visibly falls behind cities like Madrid and Seville in terms of maintaining and improving housing, urban and transport planning and lost the initiative it once held.

Dramatic and urgent action is needed in Barcelona to stop the decline, improve urban and transport planning and make Barcelona more sustainable, liveable and healthier by reducing air pollution and noise levels, heat island effects and increase green space and physical activity[3]. It is time for a radical rethink to revitalise the city and make it a city for people, rather than for cars, which it seems at the moment.

Janet Sanz, responsible for Ecology, Urbanism and Mobility in the Barcelona city council wants a Plan Cerdá for the 21st Century and asked the chief architect, Xavier Matilla, to come up with a competition proposal to get a team together to come up with a plan[4]. Here are some of the changes that I believe should be considered and made. The list is not inclusive and detailed but provides some overall ideas.

Urban and transport planning principles and actions for changes in Barcelona

1 Either improve and enlarge sustainable and healthy public transport connecting Barcelona better with rest of the metropolitan area, or spread work places and jobs more throughout the metropolitan area reducing the need for extensive mobility. Mobility is strongly related to land use and the great influx of cars from the Metropolitan area into Barcelona city.

2 Accelerate the Superillas program and create over 500 SuperIllas or something equivalent in Barcelona, which will reduce air pollution and noise levels, heat island effects and increase green space and physical activity and thereby prevent nearly 700 premature deaths each year in Barcelona[5]

3 Move towards a 15-minute city like was proposed for Paris, where work, school, entertainment and other activities are reachable within a 15-minute walk of the home[6,7]. This will require a mixing of different population groups rather than the current zoning by social economic status and therefore reduce inequalities.

4 Make any new urban development (e.g. new Forum area development) car free and with easy access to

active and public transportation. A successful examples is Vauban in Freiburg, Germany, which is neighbourhood without cars and sustainable housing[8].

5 Revitalise the old city and pedestrianize Via Laietana, Passeig de Colon and Carrer de Fontanella and connect them with the Ramblas to create a walking circle and use some of the space for things like new markets to promote local (Catalan) products. Furthermore, cover the Ronda Litoral along Passeig de Colon and create a large square opening up the space to the harbour for use of specific people´s activities.

6 Create a Rambla in each barrio in Barcelona like the Rambla de Poblenou, where people can walk and cycle and enjoy green space, and where car use is restricted. Try to the connect then the Ramblas throughout the city to create a network of ramblas.

7 Introduce and enforce 30 km/hr in all streets of Barcelona. Currently we have autopistas running through Barcelona like Calle Aragon, but lower speeds on the roads will lead to less air pollution and noise and less severe accidents[9]. In a collision between a car and a pedestrian at 30 kilometers/hour, the pedestrian has a 90% chance of surviving, at 60 km/hr this is 10%. Car speeds are already being reduced around schools in Barcelona to 20 km/hr, but[10] but this is needed elsewhere too.

8 Introduce a requirement to make all remaining motorized traffic electric within the next 10 years,

which will greatly reduce local air pollution and noise levels and CO_2 emissions. Particularly for motorbikes this should be fairly easy and there are already a large number of rentable electric ones around in the city. Use Shanghai as example, where all motorbikes are electric.

9 Encourage and incentivise teleworking, for at least a few days per week. The pandemic has shown that for many jobs teleworking is possible, which reduces the need for commuting and reduces air pollution and CO2 emissions[11].

10 Support the local economy and disencourage e-commerce. E-commerce (online buying) has been growing dramatically, but it leads to local shops closing and dead shopping streets in the long term and increased traffic and pollution in the short term because of all the (home) deliveries. Pedestrianizing streets and/or reducing car traffic are good ways to increase retail sales[12]

11 Increase green space throughout the city as it important for people´s mental health and reduces premature mortality[13,14]. There is not only a need for new developments like the park in Plaza Glories, but also more green in the streets. We need to dig up asphalt and plant more green, which will reduce heat island effects and contributes to CO2 sequestration.

12 Increase the cycling network further as a way to reduce motorised traffic and increase activity mobility and therefore increase physical activity and people´s

health[15]. Great progress has been made to create cycling lanes, but there are still gaps in the network. A cycling lane in all streets should be the aim. It will provide people with the opportunity to build physical activity into their daily lives like daily commutes, because they have often not enough time to go to the gym.

Finally, any proposals for a new Pla Cerdá should go through quantitative environmental, climate, health and equity assessments, and any changes monitored throughout and after the implementation in terms of environmental, climate, health and equity effects to optimize impacts.

In conclusion

Barcelona needs to rethink its urban and transport planning quickly and drastically to recapture the lead in urban planning that Barcelona was renowned for worldwide. Ildefonso Cerdá planned the Eixample with health in mind and Barcelona is one of the best examples of a city that planned for health. His vision of wide open streets with fresh air became large autopistas running through the city filled with health threatening air pollution. We need to go back to his original vision.

There is a lot of citizen support build up to improve the city, for example through grass root organisations like Recuperem la Ciuatat (https://www.recuperemlaciutat.com/), but also resistance from parts of society, and it is important to get everyone on board to make Barcelona more sustainable, liveable and healthier.

First published as

https://www.isglobal.org/en/healthisglobal/-/custom-blog-portlet/radical-changes-in-urban-and-transport-planning-are-needed-for-a-healthier-barcelona-the-new-plan-cerda-for-21st-century/4735173/0

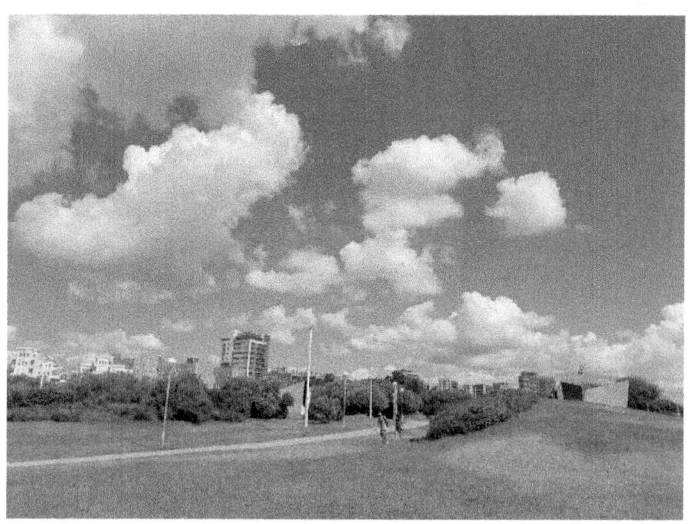

Park de Poblenou, Barcelona, Spain

10 POST-COVID19 CITIES; NEW URBAN MODELS TO MAKE CITIES HEALTHIER

"Never waste a good crisis"

The COVID19 pandemic is a wake-up call. Our world is and won´t be the same, nor will be our cities. It may be an opportunity though to build better and more sustainable societies and cities. The pandemic and the related restrictions give us time to reflect and think about solutions for the long term, while addressing an important short term problem. What kind of changes should we make to secure long term beneficial health impacts?

Cities are centres of innovation and wealth creation, but also hotspots of air pollution and noise, heat island effects and lack of green space, which are all detrimental to human health. They are also hotspots of COVID19 now. Cities are complex systems and are attractive because of the jobs, social ecosystem, events and unlimited opportunities they offer. They also have close personal contacts and large inequalities, which have become more visible with COVID19.

The noticeable visible impacts of the COVID19 pandemic are, for example, the lack of tourists, shop closures, and underused public transport in cities. The prevention measures such as hygiene (e.g. mask use) and social distancing have made us re-think how we use public space, our mode of transport and where we work (i.e. more teleworking).

One of the great challenges of cities is (suboptimal) urban and transport planning, with streets in many cities dominated by cars. For example, a city like Barcelona has some of the highest traffic density and air pollution and noise levels in Europe, which are responsible for an estimated 3000 premature deaths per year[1]. Sixty percent of public space is used by cars, while only 1 out of 4 trips is by car, and it could be used in a healthier.

During the COVD19 pandemic cities have started to push out cars, increase space for active transportation and increased their cycling lanes and rates[2,3]. During lockdowns, around 90% of car drives did not miss their commute at all or some aspects, while around 90% of cyclists missed commuting a lot or some aspects of it[4]. And air pollution and noise levels dropped considerably[5].

Therefore, is it time to re-think our urban models? In the 20th Century cities appeared to be designed for cars, but in the 21st Century, should we aim for cities for people? Should we aim for cities that are smart, sustainable, liveable, equitable and healthy, apply nature based solutions, have a circular economy and promote active mobility and green space?

New urban models

A number of new urban concepts are being introduced in various cities that go some way to address these issues like the Compact city, Superblocks, 15 Minute city, Car free city or a mixture of these. What are some of the likely impacts?

The Compact city

Compact cities are cities with higher density, shorter travel distances and higher diversity. Compared to sprawled cites their CO2 emissions are lower and they are healthier because of increased land use mix and the shorter and healthier mobility opportunities. Making cities 30% more compact could avoid around 400-800 disability adjusted life years per 100,000 people annually depending on the type of city[6,7].

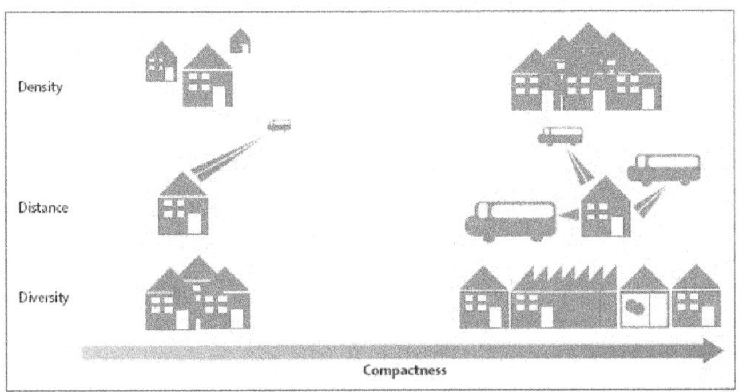

The Compact city[6]

Superblocks

Over 500 superblocks are planned in Barcelona, which reduce motorized traffic in some streets of a block and provide space for people, active travel and green space. They will reduce air pollution and noise levels, heat island effects and increase green space and physical activity and thereby could prevent nearly 700 premature deaths each year in Barcelona[8]. Similar principles are applied in low traffic neighbourhoods[9]

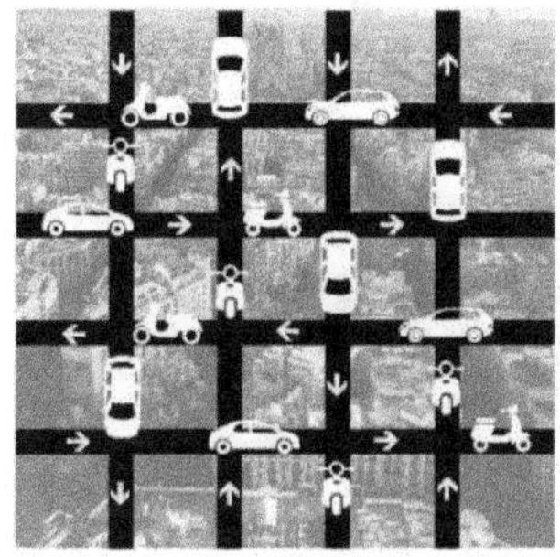
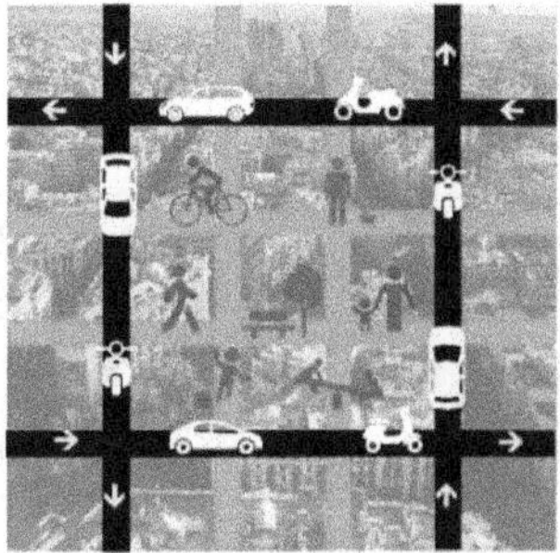

Superblock, Barcelona

The 15-minute city

Paris is introducing the 15-minute city, where work, school, entertainment and other activities are reachable within a 15-minute walk of the home[10,11]. The 15-minute city will require a fairly radical re-think of our cities and a mixing of different population groups rather than the current zoning by social economic status and therefore likely to reduce inequalities. It will also reduce the need for long distance travel and thereby CO2 emissions, and air pollution and noise levels.

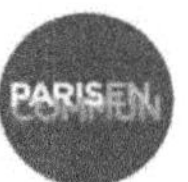

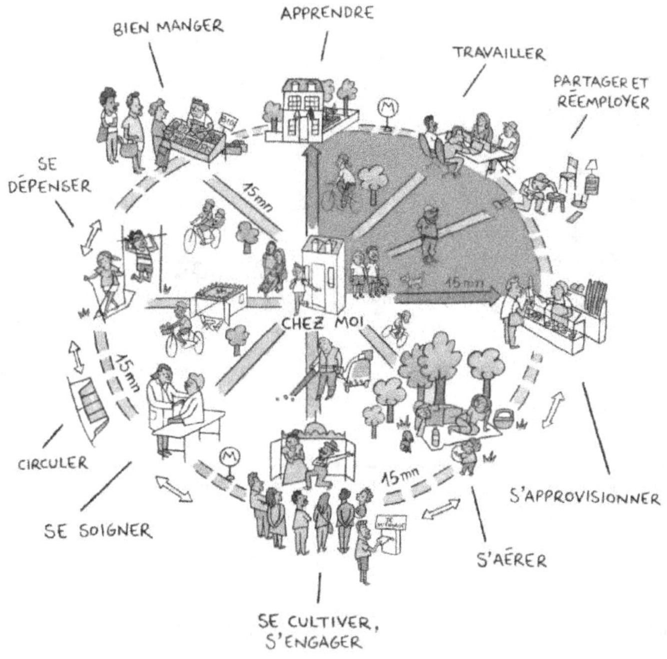

15-minute city, Paris

Hamburg plans to be car free by 2034, partly to address the climate crisis. Car free cities reduce unnecessary private motorized traffic and provide easy access to active and public transportation. They reduce air pollution and noise levels, increase physical activity and create space for green space[12]. A successful example is Vauban in Freiburg, Germany, which is neighbourhood without cars and with sustainable housing.

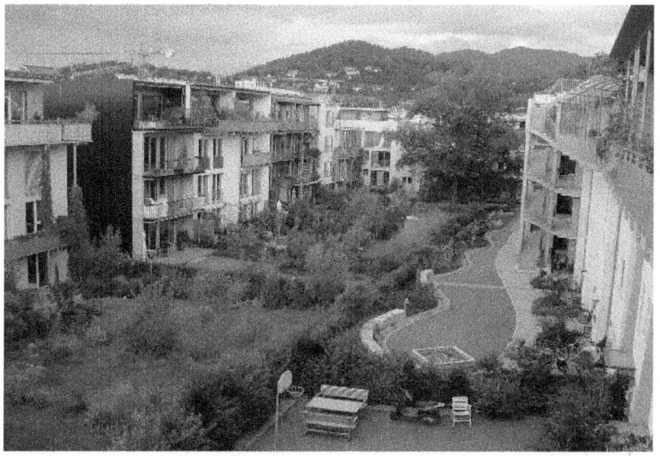

Car Free, Vauban, Freiburg, Germany

Common principles

What these new urban models have in common is that they inverse the transport planning pyramid where the priority for planning for cars is replaced by giving priority to public transportation and walking and cycling.

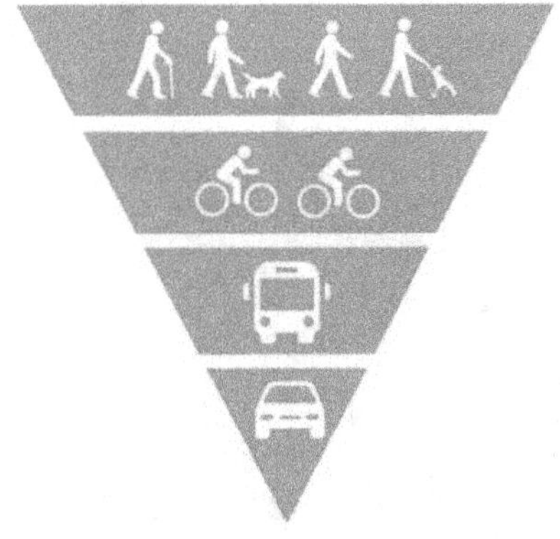

Optimal transport planning pyramid

Increasing the cycling network and thereby cycling rates is a way to reduce motorised traffic and CO2 emissions and increase active mobility and therefore increase physical activity and people´s health[13]. This will provide people with the opportunity to build physical activity into their daily lives like daily commutes, as they have often not enough time to go to the gym. Great progress has been made to create and increase cycling lanes, but they work only if they are safe and form part of a network.

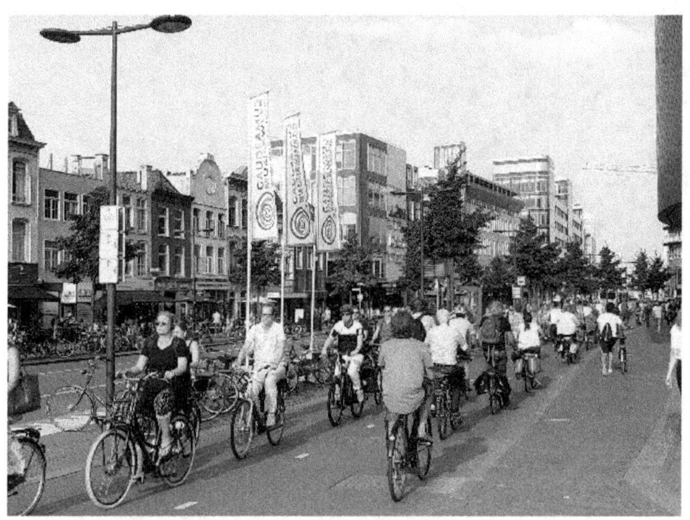

Cycling city, Utrecht, The Nethelands

What else they share to some extent is access to green space, which is important for, for example, people´s mental health, cognitive functioning and life expectancy[14,15]. There is not only a need for new developments like parks, but also more green in streets. We need to dig up asphalt and plant more trees, which will reduce heat island effects and contributes to CO2 sequestration and health[16].

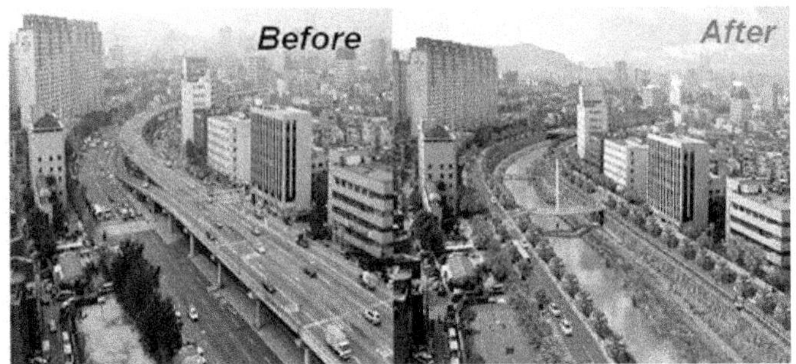

Seoul, South Korea

Recent developments

During the pandemic many people have taken to work at home (i.e teleworking), which reduces the need for commuting and reduces air pollution and CO2 emissions[17]. The question is if this trend persists, but we should encourage and incentivise teleworking, for at least a few days per week. Unfortunately, E-commerce (online buying) has been growing dramatically, and this may lead to local shops closing and dead shopping streets in the long term and increased traffic and pollution in the short term, because of all the (home) deliveries. Pedestrianizing streets and/or reducing car traffic are good ways to increase retail sales[18]. We need to support the local economy and disencourage e-commerce.

Systemic and holistic approaches, policies and investments

Cities are complex systems and to address their challenges we need systemic and holistic approaches taking into many different factors and feedback loops, and address sustainability (i.e. climate crisis), livability, health and equity simultaneously. Too often we find silos by sector in cities, which stops the implementation of these approaches that address multiple challenges. We need approaches with involvement of multiple stakeholders and disciplines[19].

One of the great challenges many cities suffer are outdated legislation e.g. zoning laws, which prevent mixed land use, which is essential for active mobility and good for health[20]. Any new legislation, including for new urban developments should include planning indicators that improve health, which is often not the case[21]. Furthermore, health impact assessments should be used to assess, which are the healthiest planning scenarios[22].

Recently the World Health Organisation published a manifesto for a healthy recovery from the COVID19, including building healthy and liveable cities[23]. These ideas need support and investments. The European Green Deal may be an opportunity. It is a comprehensive road map striving to make the EU more resource-efficient and sustainable, and a great opportunity to make cities carbon neutral, more liveable and healthier through better urban and transport planning[24].

Let us take this opportunity to make our cities better.

First published as: https://www.isglobal.org/en/healthisglobal/-/custom-blog-portlet/post-covid-19-cities-new-urban-models-to-make-cities-healthier/4735173/0

20 TRENDS FOR CITIES IN THE 20S

Early January 2020 I sat down and thought about what may be the trends for the next 10 years in cities. Most of them were already existing, but I wondered which would be the main trends. I assumed a slow progress of what was already going on. Little did I know that our world and our cities were to change dramatically because of the COVID19 pandemic. Many of the trends I thought of are still there, but the speed may change.

20 TRENDS FOR CITIES IN THE 20s

By Mark Nieuwenhuijsen, Director of the Initiative on Urban Planning, Environment and Health at ISGlobal

URBAN PLANNING

1. Urbanization continues –cities get bigger

Urbanization is continuing with up 70% of the population living in urban areas within the next 15-20 years. Employment, innovation and wealth creation continue to be the drivers for cities and the increase in their population.

2. Green is the new black

Nature based solutions such as green walls and roofs will be increasingly used in cities as a guiding principle in planning. Greening cities mitigates air pollution, noise and heat levels, and sequesters CO_2. Replacing roads and car parks with green spaces is an approach to change the environment from detrimental to beneficial for health.

3. Car free drop offs at schools

Air pollution leads to childhood asthma and slower cognitive growth, among other conditions. In the 20s we will see more active commuting of kids to school and the banning of drop offs by cars. Areas around schools will become protected areas leading to healthier and more intelligent children.

4. Buildings: taller and taller

Cities are getting bigger, but also taller with the increase in high rises in many cities, particularly in the centres. The strong competition for land means that any gaps in cities are being filled up, but there is still further sprawl at the edges of the cities. The latter will lead to longer commuting times and more congestion as public transport services are unable to keep with demands.

5. Public space to the people!

A large amount of public space is used by cars rather than by people. Pedestrians are often squeezed to the side of the road, while cars enjoy a large amount of space. A more human centric approach in cities will lead to cities for people. Safe and more aesthetically pleasing streets will lead to more activities of people in the streets.

SUSTAINABILITY

The energy transition – from a fossil fuel to renewables – is gaining pace, and cities will contribute significantly for example by reducing their emissions from transportation and improving building standards, and generating renewable energy by putting solar panels on roofs.

6. The fight towards carbon neutral and resilient cities

Cities are working harder than ever to address the climate crisis as they can feel the direct effects. Cities have a clear vision and compete with each other when to be carbon neutral: 2030, 2040, or 2050. Organisations like C40 and Global Covenant of Mayors for Climate and Energy will gain further importance.

7. Smart cities, here they are

In the 20s we will see an increase in the number of sensors to measure and better control what is going on in cities and make them more efficient. However, privacy concerns will grow and tighter regulation is required for this. Also, smarter will not only be in terms of technologies but also focus more lifestyle and behaviour choices.

8. Cleaning the air from pollution

Air pollution levels will decline in the 20s because of the well-recognized health effects: premature mortality, respiratory and cardiovascular mortality, and poor mental health, among others. Measures such as low emission zones and congestion charging are being introduced in many cities together with other measures to reduce air pollution from transport and household heating.

9. More systemic approaches and multi-disciplinarity

Economic progress, energy, mobility, climate change, and health are highly inter-related and require systematic approaches to create more sustainable, liveable and healthier cities. Traditional silos between sectors will be broken down and solutions will be found by multidisciplinary teams. Finally, cities will work harder to accomplish the Sustainable Development Goals.

MOBILITY

Cars currently take up a large amount of public space in cities while the transport mode share is much smaller.

10. To bike or not to bike: that's not a question

Cycling heavens such as The Netherlands and Denmark will become the norm rather than being the exception. Many cities have introduced bike lanes to increase the mode share of cycling, which currently is often very low. In the 20s we will see a move towards segregated cycling networks as they are the only way to increase cycling mode share.

Cycling has many advantages: it reduces disease and premature mortality, combines transport with the gym, causes less air pollution, noise and CO2 emissions, uses less public space and leads to more happiness.

11. Goal: car-free cities

Cars take up a large amount of public space in cities while the transport mode share is much smaller, and cars are parked up to 96% of the time. This public space can be used in a much better and healthier way like, for example, by trees and activity space by people.

12. Transport goes electric

The climate crisis and air pollution problems will lead to a rapid electrification of vehicles in cities in the 20s and some cities will only allow electric vehicles in the city by the end of the decade. Electric cars though won't solve all the problems in cities: still take up a lot of public space and produce non-tail air pollution and noise. Delivery vehicles are an important emissions source and will have to be electric by the end of the decade in cities.

13. Autonomous vehicles are coming

The technology for autonomous vehicles is progressing rapidly and will be introduced in cites in the 20s. This is likely to have a significant impact on urban planning and mobility, but the extent, direction and implications are hard to predict as it depends to a large extent on pricing and lifestyle choices. Furthermore, there will be other forms of autonomous platforms like delivery pods and shopping aids that require space.

14. Connecting better the metropolitan area with the city

In the 20s we will see more emphasis on providing good public transport connections and also building metropolitan (high speed) bike lanes to reduce car use and congestion. There will also be a better distribution of services and employment opportunities throughout the metropolitan area. City to city connection will become more important and increase leading to increased air travel over long distances and trains over short distances.

SOCIETY

15. Bad news: inequality increases

Due to global trends, inequality and diversity will increase in cities: they are magnets for the poor searching for employment and for the rich searching for entertainment. To some extent cities may be able to address this to providing social housing and rent control, but the impact is likely to be limited under the current economic system.

16. What runs the change? The cities.

Cities are more agile, feel any effects on citizens faster and are more responsive to the needs of people than countries. National governments have got stuck and decision making is slow because of partisan politics in some countries, the fracturing of political parties in many other countries, and the vested interest of certain groups in all countries. Cities will lead in many areas and introduce new progressive policies that directly benefit citizens.

17. People have the power!

Citizen engagement and participatory approaches will become more important as citizens will have a greater awareness of what they want in the city and how to achieve it. There will be increased involvement of the socially marginalized, to improve their living conditions, mobility and the level of their equity. Co-creation and novel co-governance are the future.

18. Global economy vs. local circular economy: David against Goliath

Cities demand almost two thirds of global energy, produce up to 80% of greenhouse gas emissions and 50% of global waste. The circular economy can provide a policy response to cope with these challenges, as a driver for economic growth, jobs and environmental quality. The attention to re-use and recycling in cities will increase, as well as the balance between what the cities get in and wat they throw out.

19. The end of the shops as we know them

Online buying will further increase at the expense of shopping in the high street and the shopping mall. Shop closures are unavoidable and may lead to a further decline of the high street and shopping mall. However, as people would like to see and meet other people there will be an increase in other facilities to meet people such as restaurants and new community centres to bring people together.

20. Health and well-being will rule city policies

Health will become the central focus point of cities. The ageing population in many cities will put restraints on some cities but also open new doors to innovations not envisaged before. Cities for the children, women and elderly adults will replace cities for the fittest. Health in all policies will be the policy framework.

First published as

https://20tendencias.isglobal.org/

EPILOQUE

The COVID19 pandemic is a dramatic event in our human history, but also provides a time of reflection. I used the time to think a bit more about how cities and citizens could react and what our cities of the future should look like through a number of short posts on blogs.

Cities are still great places to live and work and they bring people together from all ways of life. They concentrate people in some places of the world that limits the damage we do to the earth in other places. They are a relative efficient way to inhabit this world with some many people. But as I laid out they could be more sustainable, liveable and healthy with better urban and transport planning.

The COVID19 pandemic has put health at the top of the world´s agenda, something that has never been achieved by urban and transport planning and its externalities (e.g. air pollution, noise, heat islands, lack of green space and physical activity) even though over the year they have a much larger impact.

Why is this, and how can we change this and reduce health burden of our current urban and transport practices. To make changes, normally they are a number of prerequisites you need:

- Crisis
- Knowledge
- Technology
- Partnership
- Vision
- Leadership
- Funding

I believe that a number of them are in place and therefore I believe that it is time to start making changes. Of course as you seen in this book, there are cities that have already started, and the COVID19 pandemic will speed things up. But we need to go more widely and faster.

Only together we can make these changes, and in this time of reflection we should lay the ground work and advance as much of we can. We all deserve sustainable, liveable and healthy cities.

WHY DO YOU DRIVE THOUGH MY LITTLE STREET?

Calle Taulat, Poblenou, Barcelona

Because you think I like to breathe in you air pollution, listen to your noise or I cannot walk properly because you take up so much space?

I don't because I live in the street and enjoy my peace and quietness

Of course you are welcome in my street to deliver something, if you visit a shop, if you live here, or you cycle or walk through it.

The city council has put temporary valles so people on the Ramblas the Poblenou can walk without having to stop for cars. And when you drive through my street, you move them and don't put them back. You think that is alright?

Next time take a big road like Passeign de Calvell. It is not much of an effort for you but a great pleasure to me.

References

1 References

1. EPIWIN 2020. WHO Information network for epidemics. Update #18. 20-03-2020

2. Neil M Ferguson, Daniel Laydon, Gemma Nedjati-Gilani, Natsuko Imai, Kylie Ainslie, Marc Baguelin, Sangeeta Bhatia, Adhiratha Boonyasiri, Zulma Cucunubá, Gina Cuomo-Dannenburg, Amy Dighe, Ilaria Dorigatti, Han Fu, Katy Gaythorpe, Will Green, Arran Hamlet, Wes Hinsley, Lucy C Okell, Sabine van Elsland, Hayley Thompson, Robert Verity, Erik Volz, Haowei Wang, Yuanrong Wang, Patrick GT Walker, Caroline Walters, Peter Winskill, Charles Whittaker, Christl A Donnelly, Steven Riley, Azra C Ghani. Impact of non-pharmaceutical interventions (NPIs) to reduce COVID19 mortality and healthcare demand 2020 https://www.imperial.ac.uk/media/imperial-college/medicine/sph/ide/gida-fellowships/Imperial-College-COVID19-NPI-modelling-16-03-2020.pdf Accessed 14/03/2020

3. Covid19Risk (2020) https://covid-19-risk.github.io/map/ Accessed 21/03/2020

4. WEF 2020 https://www.weforum.org/agenda/2020/03/chinas-pollution-coronavirus-lockdown-covid19-enviroment/ Accessed 14/03/2020

5. Romei V and Burn-Murdoch J (2020) https://www.ft.com/content/d184fa0a-6904-11ea-800d-da70cff6e4d3 Accesed 22/03/2020

6. Space 2020 https://www.space.com/italy-coronavirus-outbreak-response-reduces-emissions-satellite-images.html Accessed 14/03/2020

7. @contaminacio_ https://twitter.com/contaminacio_ Accessed 14/03/2020

8. Watts J and Kommenda N (2020) https://www.theguardian.com/environment/2020/mar/23/coronavirus-pandemic-leading-to-huge-drop-in-air-pollution Accessed 23/03/2020

9. Lelieveld J, Pozzer A, Pöschl U, Fnais M, Haines A, Münzel T. Loss of life expectancy from air pollution compared to other risk factors: a worldwide perspective. Cardiovasc Res. 2020 Mar 3. doi: 10.1093/cvr/cvaa025.

10. GBD 2017 Risk Factor Collaborators. Global, regional, and national comparative risk assessment of 84 behavioural, environmental and occupational, and metabolic risks or clusters of risks for 195 countries and territories, 1990-2017: a systematic analysis for the Global Burden of Disease Study 2017. Lancet. 2018 Nov 10;392(10159):1923-1994

11. WHO   2020 https://en.wikipedia.org/wiki/List_of_countries_by_traffic-related_death_rate Accesed 14/03/2020

12. Costello A, Abbas M, Allen A et al. Managing the health effects of climate change: *Lancet* and University College London Institute for Global Health Commission. *Lancet.* 2009; 373: 1693-1733

13. McMahon (2020) https://www.forbes.com/sites/jeffmcmahon/2020/03/11/coronavirus-lockdown-may-save-more-lives-from-pollution-and-climate-than-from-virus/24. 20Trends. https://20trends.isglobal.org/ Accessed 14/03/2020

14. Aufhammer et al 2020 http://www.g-feed.com/2020/03/covid-19-reduces-economic-activity.html Accessed 21/03/2020

15. Barbiroglio E (2020) https://www.forbes.com/sites/emanuelabarbiroglio/2020/03/20/people-living-in-polluted-cities-are-at-higher-risk-from-covid-19/#6fe9e04a4b99 21/03/2020

16. Cui, Y., Zhang, Z., Froines, J. *et al.* Air pollution and case fatality of SARS in the People's Republic of China: an ecologic study. *Environ Health* **2**, 15 (2003). https://doi.org/10.1186/1476-069X-2-15

17. Fitbit 2020 https://blog.fitbit.com/covid-19-global-activity/

18. Wyke et aL 2020 https://docs.google.com/document/u/1/d/e/2PACX-1vR5AdOmF2effrg-lpBXtvh0stbxM0W6xTDwV2J-xlgHB8rPfZl5bLVR5eL7VV2m_W9xx5PgH26TB0vq/pub   Accessed 20/03/2020

19. Insurance journal. 2020 https://www.insurancejournal.com/news/international/2020/03/12/560943.htm. Accessed 13/03/2020

20. Parmar D, Stavropoulou C, Ioannidis JP. Health outcomes during the 2008 financial crisis in Europe: systematic literature review. BMJ. 2016 Sep 6;354:i4588.

21. Portes (2020) https://www.theguardian.com/commentisfree/2020/mar/25/there-is-no-trade-off-between-the-economy-and-health Accessed 26/03/2020

22. Bliss and Capps (2020) https://www.citylab.com/life/2020/03/coronavirus-data-cities-rural-areas-pandemic-health-risks/607783/ Accessed 20/03/2020

23. Nieuwenhuijsen M. urban and transport pathways to carbon neutral, liveable and healthy cities. Environment Int 2020 (in press)

2 References:

1. Warburton, D. E. R., Nicol, C. W. & Bredin, S. S. D. Health benefits of physical activity: The evidence. *CMAJ* vol. 174 801–809 (2006).

2. World Health Organization. Physical activity. https://www.who.int/news-room/fact-sheets/detail/physical-activity. Accessed April 20th, 2020.

3. FitBit. The Impact Of Coronavirus On Global Activity - Fitbit Blog. https://blog.fitbit.com/covid-19-global-activity/. Accessed April 20th, 2020.

4. Mobility, G. Spain March 29, 2020 Mobility changes. (2020).

5. Apple. COVID-19 - Mobility Trends Reports - Apple. https://www.apple.com/covid19/mobility. Accessed April 20th, 2020.

6. World Health Organization. WHO | Information sheet: global recommendations on physical activity for health 18 - 64 years old. *WHO* (2015).

7. Organization, W. health. WHO | Information sheet: global

recommendations on physical activity for health 65 years and above. *WHO* (2015).

8.   World Health Organization. WHO | Information sheet: global recommendations on physical activity for health 5 - 17 years old. https://www.who.int/dietphysicalactivity/publications/recommendations5_17years/en/.

9.   Pedlar, C. R. *et al.* Cardiovascular response to prescribed detraining among recreational athletes. *J. Appl. Physiol.* **124**, 813–820 (2018).

10.   Nieman, P., Leblanc, C. M. & Canadian Paediatric Society, H. A. L. and S. M. C. Psychosocial aspects of child and adolescent obesity. *Paediatr. Child Health* **17**, 205–208 (2012).

11.   Campbell, J. P. & Turner, J. E. Debunking the Myth of Exercise-Induced Immune Suppression: Redefining the Impact of Exercise on Immunological Health Across the Lifespan . *Frontiers in Immunology* vol. 9 648 (2018).

12.   Puente-Maestu, L. & Stringer, W. W. Physical activity to improve health: do not forget that the lungs benefit too. *Eur Respir J* **51**, 1702468 (2018).

13.   Hancox, R. J. & Rasmussen, F. Does physical fitness enhance lung function in children and young adults? *Eur. Respir. J.* **51**, 1701374 (2018).

14.   McDowell, C. P., Dishman, R. K., Gordon, B. R. & Herring, M. P. Physical Activity and Anxiety: A Systematic Review and Meta-analysis of Prospective Cohort Studies. *American Journal of Preventive Medicine* vol. 57 545–556 (2019).

15.   Zahl, T., Steinsbekk, S. & Wichstrøm, L. Physical Activity, Sedentary Behavior, and Symptoms of Major Depression in Middle Childhood. *Pediatrics* **139**, e20161711 (2017).

16.   Chastin, S. F. M., Palarea-Albaladejo, J., Dontje, M. L. & Skelton, D. A. Combined Effects of Time Spent in Physical Activity, Sedentary Behaviors and Sleep on Obesity and Cardio-Metabolic Health Markers: A Novel Compositional Data Analysis Approach. *PLoS One* **10**, (2015).

17.   Swift, D. L., Johannsen, N. M., Lavie, C. J., Earnest, C. P. & Church, T. S. The role of exercise and physical activity in weight loss and maintenance. *Prog. Cardiovasc. Dis.* **56**, 441–447 (2014).

18.   Shiroma, E. J. & Lee, I.-M. Physical activity and cardiovascular health: lessons learned from epidemiological studies across age, gender, and race/ethnicity. *Circulation* **122**, 743–52 (2010).

19.   Lombardi, G., Ziemann, E. & Banfi, G. Physical Activity and Bone Health: What Is the Role of Immune System? A Narrative Review of the Third Way . *Frontiers in Endocrinology* vol. 10 60 (2019).

20.   Unger, J. B. & Johnson, C. A. Social relationships and physical activity in health club members. *Am. J. Heal. Promot.* **9**, 340–343 (1995).

21.   Qian, H. *et al.* Indoor transmission of SARS-CoV-2. *medRxiv* 2020.04.04.20053058 (2020) doi:10.1101/2020.04.04.20053058.

22.   Rojas-Rueda, D., Nieuwenhuijsen, M. J., Gascon, M., Perez-Leon, D. & Mudu, P. Green spaces and mortality: a systematic review and meta-analysis of cohort studies. *Lancet Planet. Heal.* **3**, e469– e477 (2019).

23.   Gascon, M., Zijlema, W., Vert, C., White, M. P. & Nieuwenhuijsen, M. J. Outdoor blue spaces, human health and well-being: A systematic review of quantitative studies. *International Journal of Hygiene and Environmental Health* vol. 220 1207–1221 (2017).

3 References

This blog is based on the following scientific article: [1]Nieuwenhuijsen M. Urban and transport planning pathways to carbon neutral, liveable and healthy cities; a review of the current evidence. Environment International 2020 – Published April 16, 2020

4 References

1.   Khreis H, Warsow KM, Verlinghieri E, Guzman A, Pellecuer L, Ferreira A, Jones I, Heinen E, Rojas-Rueda D, Mueller N, Schepers P, Lucas K, Nieuwenhuijsen M. The health impacts of traffic-related exposures in urban areas: Understanding real effects, underlying driving forces and

co-producing future directions. Journal of Transport & Health, 2016;3:249-267

2.   Mueller N, Rojas-Rueda D, Basagaña X, Cirach M, Cole-Hunter T, Dadvand P, Donaire-Gonzalez D, Foraster M, Gascon M, Martinez D, Tonne C, Triguero-Mas M, Valentín A, Nieuwenhuijsen M. Urban and Transport Planning Related Exposures and Mortality: A Health Impact Assessment for Cities. Environ Health Perspect. 2017; 125(1):89-96

3.   ISGlobal 2019. https://www.isglobal.org/en/publication/-/asset_publisher/ljGAMKTwu9m4/content/7-maneras-en-que-las-bicicletas-pueden-hacer-las-ciudades-mas-saludables accesed 10 May 2019

4.   Dons, E., Rojas-Rueda, D., Anaya-Boig, E., Avila-Palencia, I., Brand, C., Cole-Hunter, T., ... & Kahlmeier, S. (2018). Transport mode choice and body mass index: cross-sectional and longitudinal evidence from a European-wide study. *Environment international, 119*, 109-116.

5.   Castro, Alberto, et al. "Physical activity of electric bicycle users compared to conventional bicycle users and non-cyclists: Insights based on health and transport data from an online survey in seven European cities." *Transportation research interdisciplinary perspectives* 1 (2019): 100017.

6.   Gössling S and Choi AS. Transport transitions in Copenhagen: Comparing the cost of cars and bicycles. Ecological Economics 2015; 113; 006-113

7.   Mueller N, Rojas-Rueda D, Salmon M, Martinez D, Ambros A, Brand C, de Nazelle A, Dons E, Gaupp-Berghausen M, Gerike R, Götschi T, Iacorossi F, Panis LI, Kahlmeier S, Raser E, Nieuwenhuijsen M; PASTA

consortium. Health impact assessment of cycling network expansions in European cities. Prev Med. 2018;.pii: S0091-7435(17)30497-8

8.   Nieuwenhuijsen MJ. Urban and transport planning pathways to carbon neutral, liveable and healthy cities; A review of the current evidence. Environ Int. 2020 Apr 6:105661.

5 References

1.   Nieuwenhuijsen M 2020a https://www.isglobal.org/healthisglobal/-/custom-blog-portlet/covid-19-en-las-ciudades-como-esta-afectando-la-pandemia-a-la-salud-urbana-/4735173/0

2.   Ajuntament   de   Barcelona   2020 https://ajuntament.barcelona.cat/superilles/es/noticia/mejoras-en-la-supermanzana-del-poblenou-gracias-a-las-aportaciones-vecinales Accessed 12/05/2020

3.   Nieuwenhuijsen, M. J., & Khreis, H. (2016). Car free cities: Pathway to healthy urban living. *Environment international*, *94*, 251-262.

4.   Vauban 2020 https://en.wikipedia.org/wiki/Vauban,_Freiburg

5.   Nieuwenhuijsen MJ. Urban and transport planning pathways to carbon neutral, liveable and healthy cities; A review of the current evidence. Environ Int. 2020b Apr 6:105661.

6.   Mueller N, Rojas-Rueda D, Khreis H, Cirach M, Andrés D, Ballester J, Bartoll X, Daher C, Deluca A, Echave C, Milà C, Márquez S, Palou J, Pérez K, Tonne C, Stevenson M, Rueda S, Nieuwenhuijsen M. Changing the urban design of cities for health: The superblock model. Environ Int. 2020; 134:105132

7.   Nieuwenhuijsen M 2020c https://theconversation.com/ensenanzas-del-coronavirus-8-medidas-para-hacer-ciudades-mas-habitables-y-saludables-136807

8.   ISGlobal   2019.   https://www.isglobal.org/en/publication/-/asset_publisher/ljGAMKTwu9m4/content/7-maneras-en-que-las-

bicicletas-pueden-hacer-las-ciudades-mas-saludables accesed 10 May 2019

9. Nieuwenhuijsen, M., Bastiaanssen, J., Sersli, S., Waygood, E. O. D., & Khreis, H. (2019). Implementing car-free cities: rationale, requirements, barriers and facilitators. In *Integrating Human Health into Urban and Transport Planning* (pp. 199-219). Springer, Cham.

10. O´Sullivan F 2020 https://www.citylab.com/environment/2020/02/paris-election-anne-hidalgo-city-planning-walks-stores-parks/606325/ Accesed 12/05/2020

6 References

1. Nieuwenhuijsen M 2020a https://www.isglobal.org/healthisglobal/-/custom-blog-portlet/covid-19-en-las-ciudades-como-esta-afectando-la-pandemia-a-la-salud-urbana-/4735173/0

2. Ajuntament de Barcelona 2020 https://ajuntament.barcelona.cat/superilles/es/noticia/mejoras-en-la-supermanzana-del-poblenou-gracias-a-las-aportaciones-vecinales Accessed 12/05/2020

3. Nieuwenhuijsen, M. J., & Khreis, H. (2016). Car free cities: Pathway to healthy urban living. *Environment international*, *94*, 251-262

4. Vauban 2020 https//en.wikipedia.org/wiki/Vauban,_Freiburg

5. Nieuwenhuijsen MJ. Urban and transport planning pathways to carbon neutral, liveable and healthy cities; A review of the current evidence. Environ Int. 2020b Apr 6:105661.

6. Mueller N, Rojas-Rueda D, Khreis H, Cirach M, Andrés D, Ballester J, Bartoll X, Daher C, Deluca A, Echave C, Milà C, Márquez S, Palou J, Pérez K, Tonne C, Stevenson M, Rueda S, Nieuwenhuijsen M. Changing the urban design of cities for health: The superblock model. Environ Int. 2020; 134:105132

7.   Nieuwenhuijsen M 2020c https://theconversation.com/ensenanzas-del-coronavirus-8-medidas-para-hacer-ciudades-mas-habitables-y-saludables-136807

8.   ISGlobal 2019. https://www.isglobal.org/en/publication/-/asset_publisher/ljGAMKTwu9m4/content/7-maneras-en-que-las-bicicletas-pueden-hacer-las-ciudades-mas-saludables accesed 10 May 2019

9.   Nieuwenhuijsen, M., Bastiaanssen, J., Sersli, S., Waygood, E. O. D., & Khreis, H. (2019). Implementing car-free cities: rationale, requirements, barriers and facilitators. In *Integrating Human Health into Urban and Transport Planning* (pp. 199-219). Springer, Cham.

10. O´Sullivan F 2020 https://www.citylab.com/environment/2020/02/paris-election-anne-hidalgo-city-planning-walks-stores-parks/606325/ Accesed 12/05/2020

Table Sources:

1 Barcelona: EMEF https://observatori.atm.cat/enquestes-de-mobilitat/Enquestes_ambit_ATM/EMEF/2018/Informe_publicacio_EMEF_2018.pdf

2 Madrid: https://www.crtm.es/media/712934/edm18_sintesis.pdf

3 Sevilla: https://www.sevilla.org/actualidad/blog/plan-de-movilidad-urbana-sostenible-de-sevilla/pmus-sevilla-diagnostico_v34.pdf

4 Bilbao: https://www.bilbao.eus/blogs/pmus/files/2016/10/PMUS-Plan-de-Movilidad-Urbana-Sostenible-de-Bilbao.pdf

5 Valencia: http://politicaterritorial.gva.es/documents/163211567/166352847/Pla+B%C3%A0sic+de+Mobilitat+de+l%27%C3%80rea+Metropolitana+de+Val%C3%A8ncia/b33d849c-4d19-42e9-98d4-1c859af18053

7 References

1. Gascon M, Triguero-Mas M, Martínez D, Dadvand P, Forns J, Plasència A, Nieuwenhuijsen MJ. Mental Health Benefits of Long-Term Exposure to Residential Green and Blue Spaces: A Systematic Review. Int J Environ Res Public Health. 2015;12:4354-4379

2. Google 2020 https://www.google.com/covid19/mobility/ Accessed 21/05/2020

3. WHO. (2016). *Urban green spaces and health. A review of evidence.* Copenhaguen. Retrieved from http://www.euro.who.int/__data/assets/pdf_file/0005/321971/Urban-green-spaces-and-health-review-evidence.pdf?ua=1

4. Nieuwenhuijsen MJ, Khreis H, Triguero-Mas M, Gascon M, Dadvand P. Fifty Shades of Green: Pathway to Healthy Urban Living. Epidemiology. 2017;28: 63–71

5. Coutts C and Hahn M. Green Infrastructure, Ecosystem Services, and Human Health. Int. J. Environ. Res. Public Health 2015, 12, 9768-9798

6. Dadvand P, Nieuwenhuijsen MJ, Esnaola M, Forns J, Basagaña X, Alvarez-Pedrerol M, Rivas I, López-Vicente M, De Castro Pascual M, Su J, Jerret8 t M, Querol X, Sunyer J. Green spaces and cognitive development in primary schoolchildren. Proc Natl Acad Sci 2015;112(26):7937-42

7. Preuß M, Nieuwenhuijsen M, Marquez S, Cirach M, Dadvand P, Triguero-Mas M, Gidlow C, Grazuleviciene R, Kruize H, Zijlema W. Low Childhood Nature Exposure is Associated with Worse Mental Health in Adulthood. Int J Environ Res Public Health. 2019 May 22;16(10). pii: E1809.

8. Kondo MC, Mueller N, Locke DH, Roman LA, Rojas-Rueda D, Schinasi LH, Gascon M, Nieuwenhuijsen MJ. Health impact assessment of Philadelphia's 2025 tree canopy cover goals. Lancet Planet Health. 2020 Apr;4(4):e149-e157.

9. Nieuwenhuijsen MJ. Urban and transport planning pathways to carbon neutral, liveable and healthy cities; A review of the current evidence. Environ Int. 2020 Apr 6:105661.

10. Ajuntament de Barcelona 2020 https://ajuntament.barcelona.cat/superilles/es/noticia/mejoras-en-

la-supermanzana-del-poblenou-gracias-a-las-aportaciones-vecinales
Accessed 12/05/2020

11. Mueller N, Rojas-Rueda D, Khreis H, Cirach M, Andrés D, Ballester J,
     Bartoll X, Daher C, Deluca A, Echave C, Milà C, Márquez S, Palou J,
     Pérez K, Tonne C, Stevenson M, Rueda S, Nieuwenhuijsen M.
     Changing the urban design of cities for health: The superblock model.
     Environ Int. 2020; 134:105132

12. Gascon M, Zijlema W, Vert C, White MP, Nieuwenhuijsen MJ. Outdoor
     blue spaces, human health and well-being: A systematic review of
     quantitative studies. Int J Hyg Environ Health. 2017; S1438-
     4639(17)30269-9.

8 References

1. Hamer, M., Kivimäki, M., Gale, C. R., & Batty, G. D. (2020). Lifestyle
    risk factors, inflammatory mechanisms, and COVID-19 hospitalization:
    A community-based cohort study of 387,109 adults in UK. *Brain,
    Behavior, and Immunity*.

2. Leandro, C. G., e Silva, W. T. F., & Lima-Silva, A. E. (2020). Covid-19
    and Exercise-Induced Immunomodulation. *Neuroimmunomodulation*,
    1.

3. Simpson, R. J., & Katsanis, E. (2020). The immunological case for
    staying active during the COVID-19 pandemic. *Brain, behavior, and
    immunity*.

4. Gascon M, Triguero-Mas M, Martínez D, Dadvand P, Forns J, Plasència
    A, Nieuwenhuijsen MJ. Mental Health Benefits of Long-Term Exposure
    to Residential Green and Blue Spaces: A Systematic Review. Int J
    Environ Res Public Health. 2015;12:4354-4379

5. Sanchez 2020
    https://www.lavanguardia.com/comer/tendencias/20200724/27077/
    platano-bloquea-entrada-celular-virus-covid-19.html

6. Restrepo (2020) https://nakedfoodmagazine.com/health-status-
    covid-19/

7. WHO 2020 https://www.who.int/publications/i/item/contact-tracing-in-the-context-of-covid-19

8. Weiss (2020) https://www.bloomberg.com/news/articles/2020-07-04/bicycles-are-pushing-aside-cars-on-europe-s-city-streets?cmpid=BBD070620_CITYLAB&utm_medium=email&utm_source=newsletter&utm_term=200706&utm_campaign=citylabdaily

9. Nieuwenhuijsen (2020) https://theconversation.com/pueden-las-ciudades-espanolas-prescindir-del-coche-139482

10. Wu, X., Nethery, R. C., Sabath, B. M., Braun, D., & Dominici, F. (2020). Exposure to air pollution and COVID-19 mortality in the United States. *medRxiv*.

11. Morawska, L., Tang, J. W., Bahnfleth, W., Bluyssen, P. M., Boerstra, A., Buonanno, G., ... & Wierzbicka, A. (2020). How can airborne transmission of COVID-19 indoors be minimised?. Environment International Volume 142, September 2020, 105832

Further reading

https://www.theguardian.com/us-news/2020/jul/24/coronavirus-smoking-cigarettes-danger-covid-19

https://www.bbc.com/news/health-53532228?utm_source=Global%20Health%20NOW%20Main%20List&utm_campaign=32c5372547-EMAIL_CAMPAIGN_2020_07_24_02_02&utm_medium=email&utm_term=0_8d0d062dbd-32c5372547-860663

9 References

1. Mueller N, Rojas-Rueda D, Basagaña X, Cirach M, Cole-Hunter T, Dadvand P, Donaire-Gonzalez D, Foraster M, Gascon M, Martinez D, Tonne C, Triguero-Mas M, Valentín A, Nieuwenhuijsen M. Urban and Transport Planning Related Exposures and Mortality: A Health Impact Assessment for Cities. Environ Health Perspect. 2017; 125(1):89-96

2.   Angulo 2020
     https://www.lavanguardia.com/local/barcelona/20200901/48325584
     0896/barcelona-restricciones-coches.html

3.   Nieuwenhuijsen MJ. Urban and transport planning pathways to carbon
     neutral, liveable and healthy cities; A review of the current evidence.
     Environ Int. 2020 Apr 6:105661.

4.   Mumbrú (2020) https://www.ara.cat/societat/Janet-Sanz-Farem-
     Cerda-XXI_0_2518548165.html

5.   Mueller N, Rojas-Rueda D, Khreis H, Cirach M, Andrés D, Ballester J,
     Bartoll X, Daher C, Deluca A, Echave C, Milà C, Márquez S, Palou J,
     Pérez K, Tonne C, Stevenson M, Rueda S, Nieuwenhuijsen M.
     Changing the urban design of cities for health: The superblock model.
     Environ Int. 2020; 134:105132

6.   Moreno 2019 http://www.moreno-web.net/the-15-minutes-city-for-
     a-new-chrono-urbanism-pr-carlos-moreno/

7.   Sisson 2020 https://www.bloomberg.com/news/articles/2020-07-
     15/mayors-tout-the-15-minute-city-as-covid-
     recovery?cmpid=BBD071620_CITYLAB&utm_medium=email&utm_so
     urce=newsletter&utm_term=200716&utm_campaign=citylabdaily

8.   Nieuwenhuijsen, M. J., & Khreis, H. (2016). Car free cities: Pathway to
     healthy urban living. *Environment international*, *94*, 251-262.

9.   Grundy C, Steinbach R, Edwards P, Green J, Armstrong B, Wilkinson P.
     Effect of 20 mph traffic speed zones on road injuries in London, 1986-
     2006: controlled interrupted time series analysis. *BMJ*.
     2009;339:b4469. Published 2009 Dec 10. doi:10.1136/bmj.b4469

10. Montilla (2020)
     https://www.lavanguardia.com/local/barcelona/20200728/48256988
     8471/colau-sanz-escoles-protegim-grevol-peaton-20kmh.html

11. Casale 2020 https://therevelator.org/telework-environmental-
     benefits/

12. Lawlor, E., 2014. The pedestrian pound. The Business Case for Better
     Streets and Places

https://www.livingstreets.org.uk/media/3890/pedestrian-pound-2018.pdf - looks like there was an update in 2018.

13. Gascon M, Triguero-Mas M, Martínez D, Dadvand P, Forns J, Plasència A, Nieuwenhuijsen MJ. Mental Health Benefits of Long-Term Exposure to Residential Green and Blue Spaces: A Systematic Review. Int J Environ Res Public Health. 2015;12:4354-4379

14. Kondo MC, Mueller N, Locke DH, Roman LA, Rojas-Rueda D, Schinasi LH, Gascon M, Nieuwenhuijsen MJ. Health impact assessment of Philadelphia's 2025 tree canopy cover goals. Lancet Planet Health. 2020 Apr;4(4):e149-e157.

15. Mueller N, Rojas-Rueda D, Salmon M, Martinez D, Ambros A, Brand C, de Nazelle A, Dons E, Gaupp-Berghausen M, Gerike R, Götschi T, Iacorossi F, Panis LI, Kahlmeier S, Raser E, Nieuwenhuijsen M; PASTA consortium. Health impact assessment of cycling network expansions in European cities. Prev Med. 2018;.pii: S0091-7435(17)30497-8

10 References

1. Mueller N, Rojas-Rueda D, Salmon M, Martinez D, Ambros A, Brand C, de Nazelle A, Dons E, Gaupp-Berghausen M, Gerike R, Götschi T, Iacorossi F, Panis LI, Kahlmeier S, Raser E, Nieuwenhuijsen M; PASTA consortium. Health impact assessment of cycling Mueller N, Rojas-Rueda D, Basagaña X, Cirach M, Cole-Hunter T, Dadvand P, Donaire-Gonzalez D, Foraster M, Gascon M, Martinez D, Tonne C, Triguero-Mas M, Valentín A, Nieuwenhuijsen M. Urban and Transport Planning Related Exposures and Mortality: A Health Impact Assessment for Cities. Environ Health Perspect. 2017; 125(1):89-96

2. Weis 2020 https://www.bloomberg.com/news/articles/2020-07-04/bicycles-are-pushing-aside-cars-on-europe-s-city-streets?cmpid=BBD070620_CITYLAB&utm_medium=email&utm_source=newsletter&utm_term=200706&utm_campaign=citylabdaily

3. Vandy (2020) https://www.bbc.com/news/world-europe-54353914

4. Rubin, O., Nikolaeva, A., Nello-Deakin, S., & te Brömmelstroet, M., (2020). What can we learn from the COVID-19 pandemic about how people experience working from home and commuting? Centre for Urban Studies, University of Amsterdam. Available at:

https://urbanstudies.uva.nl/content/blog-series/covid-19- pandemic-working-from-home-and-commuting.html

5.   Copernicus (2020)
      https://www.euronews.com/2020/08/31/european-cities-race-to-clean-the-air

6.   Stevenson, M., Thompson, J., de Sá, T. H., Ewing, R., Mohan, D., McClure, R., ... & Wallace, M. (2016). Land use, transport, and population health: estimating the health benefits of compact cities. *The lancet, 388*(10062), 2925-2935.

7.   Wikipedia (2020) https://en.wikipedia.org/wiki/Compact_city

8.   Mueller N, Rojas-Rueda D, Khreis H, Cirach M, Andrés D, Ballester J, Bartoll X, Daher C, Deluca A, Echave C, Milà C, Márquez S, Palou J, Pérez K, Tonne C, Stevenson M, Rueda S, Nieuwenhuijsen M. Changing the urban design of cities for health: The superblock model. Environ Int. 2020; 134:105132

9.   LLS (2020) https://londonlivingstreets.com/low-traffic-liveable-neighbourhoods/

10.   Moreno 2019 http://www.moreno-web.net/the-15-minutes-city-for-a-new-chrono-urbanism-pr-carlos-moreno/

11.   Sisson 2020 https://www.bloomberg.com/news/articles/2020-07-15/mayors-tout-the-15-minute-city-as-covid-recovery?cmpid=BBD071620_CITYLAB&utm_medium=email&utm_source=newsletter&utm_term=200716&utm_campaign=citylabdaily

12.   Nieuwenhuijsen, M. J., & Khreis, H. (2016). Car free cities: Pathway to healthy urban living. *Environment international, 94*, 251-262.

13.   Mueller N, Rojas-Rueda D, Salmon M, Martinez D, Ambros A, Brand C, de Nazelle A, Dons E, Gaupp-Berghausen M, Gerike R, Götschi T, Iacorossi F, Panis LI, Kahlmeier S, Raser E, Nieuwenhuijsen M; PASTA consortium. Health impact assessment of cycling network expansions in European cities. Prev Med. 2018;.pii: S0091-7435(17)30497-8

14.   Gascon M, Triguero-Mas M, Martínez D, Dadvand P, Forns J, Plasència A, Nieuwenhuijsen MJ. Mental Health Benefits of Long-Term Exposure to Residential Green and Blue Spaces: A Systematic Review. Int J Environ Res Public Health. 2015;12:4354-4379

15. Kondo MC, Mueller N, Locke DH, Roman LA, Rojas-Rueda D, Schinasi LH, Gascon M, Nieuwenhuijsen MJ. Health impact assessment of Philadelphia's 2025 tree canopy cover goals. Lancet Planet Health. 2020 Apr;4(4):e149-e157.

16. Nieuwenhuijsen MJ, Khreis H, Triguero-Mas M, Gascon M, Dadvand P. Fifty Shades of Green: Pathway to Healthy Urban Living. Epidemiology. 2017a;28: 63–71

17. Casale 2020 https://therevelator.org/telework-environmental-benefits/

18. Lawlor, E., 2014. The pedestrian pound. The Business Case for Better Streets and Places https://www.livingstreets.org.uk/media/3890/pedestrian-pound-2018.pdf - looks like there was an update in 2018.

19. Nieuwenhuijsen MJ. Urban and transport planning pathways to carbon neutral, liveable and healthy cities; A review of the current evidence. Environ Int. 2020 Apr 6:105661.

20. Nieuwenhuijsen MJ. Influence of urban and transport planning and the city environment on cardiovascular disease. Nat Rev Cardiol. 2018; 15(7):432-438

21. Mueller N, Carolyn Daher C, Rojas-Rueda D, Delgado L, Vicioso H, Gascon M, Marquet O, Vert C, Martin I, Mark Nieuwenhuijsen M. Integrating health indicators into urban and transport planning: a narrative literature review and participatory process. Env Res (submitted)

22. Nieuwenhuijsen MJ, Khreis H, Verlinghieri E, Mueller N, Rojas-Rueda D. Participatory quantitative health impact assessment of urban and transport planning in cities: A review and research needs. Environ Int. 2017b Apr 4. pii: S0160-4120(17)30128-9.

23. WHO (2020). https://www.who.int/news-room/feature-stories/detail/who-manifesto-for-a-healthy-recovery-from-covid-19

24. European Commission. Communication From The Commission To The European Parliament, The European Council, The Council, The European Economic And Social Committee And The Committee Of The Regions. The European Green Deal. Bussels, 11.12.2019. https://eur-lex.europa.eu/legal-

content/EN/TXT/HTML/?uri=CELEX:52019DC0640&from=EN (last accessed July 27, 2020)

Further reading
Nieuwenhuijsen MJ and Khreis H. (2018) Integrating health into urban and transport planning. Springer. ISBN 978-3-319-74982-2